Modern Medical Statistics

To my wife, Mary-Elizabeth

Modern Medical Statistics

A Practical Guide

Brian S. Everitt
Institute of Psychiatry, King's College London

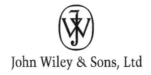

John Wiley & Sons, Ltd

First published in Great Britain in 2003 by
Arnold, a member of the Hodder Headline Group,
338 Euston Road, London NW1 3BH

Distributed in the United States of America by
Oxford University Press Inc.,
198 Madison Avenue, New York, NY10016

John Wiley & Sons Ltd, The Atrium, Southern Gate, Chichester, West
Sussex, PO19 8SQ, United Kingdom

For details of our global editorial offices, for customer services and
for information about how to apply for permission to reuse the copyright
material in this book please see our website at www.wiley.com.

British Library Cataloguing in Publication Data
A catalogue record for this book is available from the British Library

Library of Congress Cataloging-in-Publication Data
A catalog record for this book is available from the Library of Congress

ISBN: 978-0-470-71116-3

1 2 3 4 5 6 7 8 9 10

Typeset in 10/11 pt Times by Charon Tec Pvt, India

Contents

Preface

Statistical science plays an important role in medical research. Medical journals are full of statistical material, and it is increasingly common to see statistical results from research papers quoted in promotional materials for drugs and other medical therapies. Clearly clinicians and medical researchers need to know some statistics, even if only to make their discussion with a friendly statistician more fruitful. For the basic techniques such as simple inference, regression, correlation and analysis of variance, such people are well catered for by a number of excellent introductory medical statistics texts, including Altman (1991), Bland (2000) and Campbell and Machin (1999). But there have, over the last two decades or so, been advances in a number of branches of statistics that are of particular relevance to research investigations in medicine and which are not described routinely in current medical statistics texts. Many of these more recent developments are now regularly finding their way into the medical literature. It is hoped that this text will provide a useful guide and introduction to a number of these newer methods, particularly for medical researchers who, whilst not statisticians, do have a relatively firm grounding in the basics of statistics. Of course, not all methods that might come under the heading 'modern medical statistics' are included in the book. (And, of course, 'modern' is a somewhat relative term.) The choice of which methods to include and which to exclude largely reflects my own areas of interest and competence (although readers will need to assess whether the latter criterion was applied realistically). Two very obvious omissions are *neural networks* and *data mining*. Both are fashionable and may also have become respectable. But I think the jury remains out on whether they really have a great deal to offer the majority of researchers handling medical data. Perhaps in a second edition (there seems no harm in a bit of possibly wildly optimistic speculation) the issues around such methods will have been resolved, and the two topics may not even need to be mentioned; alternatively, the new edition will have to contain at least two extra chapters – we will have to wait and see.

Methods are described in a largely non-technical fashion, the emphasis instead being on examples and applications. (A small glossary included at the end of the book defines some of the terms that are mentioned only in passing in the body of the text.) Exercises are provided at the end of each chapter to allow readers to try out what has been learnt in the chapter. These exercises also make the book useful for students on applied medical statistics courses. (Solutions to some of the exercises are provided in Appendix B.)

Most of the methods of analysis included in this text can only be applied routinely with the aid of computers and statistical software. Consequently, at the end of each chapter is a section that very briefly describes software relevant to the particular techniques covered in the chapter.

My thanks are due to Ms Harriet Meteyard for her usual efficient word-processing and general support during the writing of this book, to my colleagues Sophia Rabe-Hesketh, Sabine Landau and Rebecca Walwyn, who were each kind enough to read through the manuscript and make many helpful suggestions that led to improvements, and to Dr Liz Gooster of Arnold whose comments about how to structure the book were extremely useful. In addition, I would like to express my gratitude to Mark Segal, David Spiegelhulter and Cyrus Mehta for allowing me to reproduce accounts of particular techniques from their own publications.

B.S. EVERITT
London, 2002

Prologue

A good place to begin a book dealing with the use of statistical methods in medical research is to ask why statistics is important in medicine. Here are some possible answers:

- Medical practice and medical research generate large amounts of data. Such data are generally full of uncertainty and variation, and extracting the 'signal' from the 'noise' is usually not trivial.
- Medicine involves asking questions that have strong statistical aspects. How common is the disease? Who is especially likely to contract a particular condition? What are the chances of a patient recently diagnosed with breast cancer surviving more than five years?
- The evaluation of competing treatments or preventative measures relies heavily on statistical concepts in both the design and analysis phase.

Statistics is prevalent in the medical world, but it is probably true that many clinicians and applied medical researchers regard the subject as a necessary evil. Indeed, it may be true that for many, 'statistics are numbers to which complex mathematical formulae can be applied to produce conclusions of dubious veracity and from which all wit and human life is ingenuously excluded' (Le Fanu, 1999).

It appears that the feeling of most medical researchers is that the creative ideas of medicine arise from the basic biological sciences, and that the paraphernalia of statistics has largely a control function, although they might be ready to admit that this control – implemented, for example, by means of clinical trials and epidemiology – is necessary. Statisticians, however, would probably suggest that there is a symbiotic relationship between biology and statistics in the medical field. The knowledge gained from basic biological research is only likely to be of practical value in medicine if it can be tested and confirmed in clinical and epidemiological trials. Understanding biological mechanisms in the laboratory is not usually sufficient to lead to definitive conclusions regarding the effect of a treatment or preventative measure. The biology of the organism is complex and, for example, taking a certain pill every day does not necessarily give the effect that was suggested in the laboratory. There are numerous examples of medical studies that give unexpected results. An example is given by Waldo *et al.* (1996) involving the use of d-sotalol versus placebo after infarction. The active treatment was supposed to prevent arrhythmias that could lead to sudden death, but was actually shown in the clinical trial to increase mortality.

And statisticians might point out that the major change in clinical investigation in the last hundred years or so has been the rise in quantitative reasoning – *medical statistics*. From William Farr questioning the reasons for the yawning gap in child-hood mortality rates between the rich and poor, and Florence Nightingale presenting massive amounts of data, carefully arranged and tabulated, to convince ministers, viceroys and Parliamentary commissionaires of the truth of her cause, to Austin Bradford Hill discovering the connection between smoking and lung cancer, statisticians can point to many definite success stories of statistics. Indeed, they might go even further and suggest that statistical enquiry, by determining the underlying causes of ill health such as poor sanitation, provides the means for the prevention of disease on a massive scale; consequently, statisticians have potentially a greater effect in improving human health than any number of clinicians honing their bedside technique in hospitals the world over.

It seems clear that this numerical emphasis in the medical field will continue into the next decade or longer, a situation that many clinicians have accepted and even wel-comed, as witnessed in the evidence-based medicine movement. Statistics now per-vades every aspect of medicine: hospital utility statistics, audit, resource allocation, vaccination uptake, numbers of new cases of AIDS and so on. Introductory statistics courses for doctors are widespread and generally fully subscribed, and medical jour-nals increasingly have a statistician on their editorial boards. One of the consequences of the latter move has been a more ready acceptance of the use of relatively complex and sophisticated statistical procedures in the papers published in such journals. Perhaps the most striking illustration of this point is the dramatic growth in the use of logistic regression. This technique was rarely used in epidemiology and public health research before the late 1960s. But by the end of the 1990s almost one paper in three in two respected journals, the *American Journal of Epidemiology* and the *American Journal of Public Health*, included an application of logistic regression, as shown in Figure 0.1. The reasons for the increase are: first, that the technique meets a need in

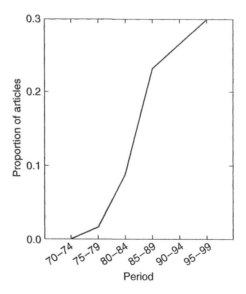

Figure 0.1 Growth in logistic regression use assessed in two major psychiatric journals. (*Source*: Levy and Stolte, 2000.)

medical research as a way of dealing with dichotomous endpoints such as incidence, prevalence and occurrence of improvement following an intervention; and second, that the calculations involved in applying the method no longer present any problems because of the wide availability of both powerful statistical software packages and relatively cheap computing in the form of the ubiquitous PC.

Logistic regression is an example of a non-trivial piece of statistical methodology that is now widely (and, on the whole, sensibly) applied by medical researchers who are not statisticians, because over the years the technique has found its way into the courses attended by such researchers. Unfortunately, many other recently developed statistical procedures that are potentially of considerable relevance in medicine have not usually been included in such courses; they are only described in the type of technical monograph or paper that most clinicians and their associates would think at least twice about reading. This is a great shame since a number of the new techniques are very powerful and can be used routinely because they have been implemented in some statistical package. Which brings us conveniently to my aim for this book: it is to introduce numerate medical researchers with a reasonable background in statistics to a range of newer methods, concentrating not on their full technical detail, but more on their practical possibilities. In this way it is hoped that the book will help in making the use of these methods more widespread in medical research.

1

The Generalized Linear Model

1.1 Introduction

The *generalized linear model* (GLM), a unified framework for regression models, has now been around for thirty years, so readers might reasonably question why it is making an appearance in the first chapter of a book dealing with 'modern' medical statistics. One rather feeble excuse is that it provides a convenient stepping-off point for the rest of the book, by covering some techniques likely to be reasonably well known to the reader, but within a framework with which they may not be entirely familiar. And GLMs are not usually described in introductory texts on medical statistics.

The term 'generalized linear model' was first introduced in a landmark paper by Nelder and Wedderburn (1972), in which a wide range of seemingly disparate problems of statistical modelling and inference (analysis of variance, analysis of covariance, multiple regression, logistic regression etc.) were set in an elegant unifying framework of great power and flexibility. A comprehensive technical account of the model is given in McCullagh and Nelder (1989), with a more concise description being available in Dobson (2001) or Cook (1998).

1.2 The generalized linear model – a brief non-technical account

The term 'regression' was first introduced by Galton in the nineteenth century to characterize a tendency towards mediocrity, that is, towards the average, observed in the offspring of children. Today regression analysis of one form or another is the mainstay of much of the analysis of medical data carried out daily. In essence, all forms of regression have as their aim the development and assessment of a mathematical model of the relationship between a *response variable*, y, and a set of q *explanatory variables* (sometimes confusingly referred to as independent variables), $x_1, x_2, \ldots, x_q$. Multiple linear regression, for example, involves the following model for y:

$$y = \beta_0 + \beta_1 x_1 + \beta_2 x_2 + \cdots + \beta_q x_q + \varepsilon \tag{1.1}$$

where $\beta_0, \beta_1, \ldots, \beta_q$ are regression coefficients that have to be estimated from sample data and ε is an error term that is assumed normally distributed with zero mean and variance σ^2. (Analysis of variance is essentially exactly the same model with $x_1, \ldots, x_q$ being dummy variables coding factor levels and interaction between factors; analysis of covariance is also the same model with a mixture of continuous and categorical explanatory variables.)

An equivalent way of writing the multiple regression model in (1.1) is as

$$y \sim N(\mu, \sigma^2) \tag{1.2}$$

where $\mu = \beta_0 + \beta_1 x_1 + \cdots + \beta_q x_q$. This makes it clear that this model is only suitable for continuous response variables with, conditional on the values of the explanatory variables, a normal distribution with constant variance.

In medical research, response variables that are neither continuous nor normally distributed are common. The most obvious examples are binary responses such as improved/not improved or dead/alive. Once again the objective is to model the mean of the relevant distribution (μ) as in multiple linear regression, but now this must be done indirectly via the use of a transformation. In a GLM this is done through the introduction of a *link function*, g, leading to the model

$$g(\mu) = \beta_0 + \beta_1 x_1 + \cdots + \beta_q x_q \tag{1.3}$$

The distribution of the response variable around its mean (often referred to as the *error distribution*) must also now be generalized, usually in a way that fits naturally with a particular link function. The result is a very wide class of regression models.

The generalization achieved by the use of (1.3) can be illustrated with *logistic regression*, a technique widely used in medical research to study the relationship between a binary response and a set of explanatory variables of interest. The expected or average value of a binary response is simply the probability of the response variable having the category coded '1' (generally the occurrence of the event of interest), say p. Modelling this directly as a linear function of explanatory variables, as is done in multiple linear regression, is clearly not sensible since it could result in fitted values of the response probability outside the range (0, 1). Instead a suitable transformation of the expected value is modelled, with the link function, g, in this case being the *logistic* or *logit* function of p, giving the model

$$\text{logit}[p] = \beta_0 + \beta_1 x_1 + \cdots + \beta_q x_q \tag{1.4}$$

that is,

$$\log \frac{p}{1-p} = \beta_0 + \beta_1 x_1 + \cdots + \beta_q x_q \tag{1.5}$$

The logistic link function is most generally associated with data having a *binomial distribution*, in which case the estimated regression coefficients may be interpreted as *log odds ratios*, as we shall illustrate in later examples. (In particular contexts, other link functions may be adopted for binary responses – see Cook, 1998, for details.)

In addition to the link function and the associated error distribution (which is assumed to be a member of a class of distributions known as the *exponential family*), a further fundamental component of a GLM is the *variance function* that captures how the variance of the response variable depends upon the mean. In many applications this aspect of such models need be of little concern to most users; it does become of importance, however, in particular circumstances that we shall illustrate in Section 1.5.

Estimation of the parameters in a GLM is usually achieved through a *maximum likelihood* approach. Details are given in McCullagh and Nelder (1989) and Cook (1998). Having estimated a GLM for some data, the question of the quality of its fit arises. Clearly the researcher needs to be satisfied that the chosen model describes the data adequately, before drawing conclusions about the parameter estimates themselves. In practice, most interest will lie in comparing the fit of competing models, particularly in the context of selecting subsets of explanatory variables that describe the data adequately. In GLMs a measure of fit is provided by a quantity known as the *deviance*. This is essentially a statistic which measures how closely the model-based fitted values of the response approximate the observed values; the deviance values quoted in this text are actually -2 times the maximized log-likelihood for a model, and differences in the deviances of competing models give a *likelihood ratio test* for comparing the models. More details of the deviance statistic are given in Cook (1998).

In the next section we describe some applications of the GLM, and show how deviance is used in practice.

1.3   Examples of the application of generalized linear models

In this section we shall describe a number of applications of GLMs and how to interpret and assess the results obtained.

1.3.1   Patients with hypertension

The data shown in Table 1.1 arise from a simple random sample of 20 patients with hypertension (Daniel, 1995). The response variable and explanatory variables are as follows:

y: mean arterial blood pressure (mmHg) – *bp*
x_1: age (years) – *age*
x_2: weight (kg) – *weight*
x_3: body surface area (m^2) – *ba*

Table 1.1   Data for 20 patients with hypertension

	bp	age	weight	ba	timeht	pulse	stress
1	105	47	85.4	1.75	5.1	63	33
2	115	49	94.2	2.10	3.8	70	14
3	116	49	95.3	1.98	8.2	72	10
4	117	50	94.7	2.01	5.8	73	99
5	112	51	89.4	1.89	7.0	72	95
6	121	48	99.5	2.25	9.3	71	10
7	121	49	99.8	2.25	2.5	69	42
8	110	47	90.9	1.90	6.2	66	8
9	110	49	89.2	1.83	7.1	69	62
10	114	48	92.7	2.07	5.6	64	35
11	114	47	94.4	2.07	5.3	74	90
12	115	49	94.1	1.98	5.6	71	21
13	114	50	91.6	2.05	10.2	68	47
14	106	45	87.1	1.92	5.6	67	80
15	125	52	101.3	2.19	10.0	76	98
16	114	46	94.5	1.98	7.4	69	95
17	106	46	87.0	1.87	3.6	62	18
18	113	46	94.5	1.90	4.3	70	12
19	110	48	90.5	1.88	9.0	71	99
20	122	56	95.7	2.09	7.0	75	99

Source: Daniel (1995).

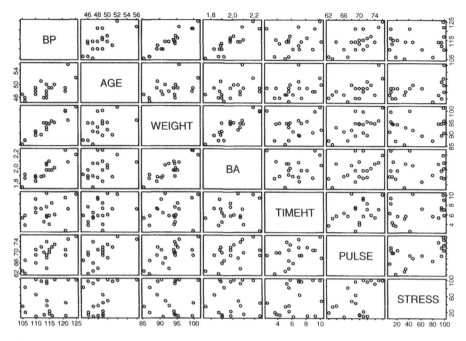

Figure 1.1   Scatterplot matrix of variables in the hypertension data.

x_4: duration of hypertension (years) – *timeht*
x_5: basal pulse (beats/min) – *pulse*
x_6: measure of stress – *stress*

(The number of observations relative to the number of variables is clearly not adequate for any convincing conclusions to be drawn from an analysis of these data, but they will serve the purpose of illustrating some features of generalized linear modelling.)

It is usually good practice to study some graphical representation of the data prior to formal modelling, and here a useful plot is provided by the *scatterplot matrix*, a grid of the scattergrams of each pair of variables (see Everitt and Dunn, 2001, for details). The diagram is shown in Figure 1.1. The plot suggests that blood pressure is most closely related to age and weight, and also indicates that several of the explanatory variables are related. There is no evidence of any outliers in the data that may distort the model fitting process.

Another useful diagram for informally examining the associations between the response variable and the explanatory variables is shown in Figure 1.2. Here blood pressure is stratified separately by values of the other variables. This diagram again suggests perhaps that weight and age are likely to be important predictors of blood pressure although the numbers of observations on which this suggestion is based are small.

For these data the response variable is continuous and we shall apply the multiple linear regression model, that is, a GLM with an identity link function and normal error terms. The results of the model fitting process are shown in Table 1.2. The estimated regression coefficients, their standard errors and associated 'z statistics' (estimate divided by standard error) should be familiar to readers from their previous experience

Mean of BP

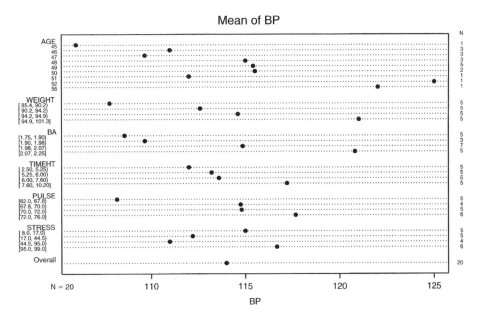

Figure 1.2 Blood pressure stratified separately by values of other variables.

Table 1.2 Results from fitting a multiple regression model to the hypertension data in Table 1.1

Covariates	Estimated regression coefficient	Standard error	Estimate/SE
Intercept	−12.870	2.557	−5.034
Age	0.703	0.050	14.177
Weight	0.970	0.063	15.369
Ba	3.776	1.580	2.390
Timeht	0.068	0.048	1.411
Pulse	−0.084	0.052	−1.637
Stress	0.006	0.003	1.633

(Dispersion parameter for Gaussian family taken to be 0.1658.)
Null deviance: 560 on 19 degrees of freedom.
Residual deviance: 2.16 on 13 degrees of freedom.

with multiple regression. It appears that age and weight are the most important predictors of blood pressure amongst patients suffering from hypertension, although this would need more detailed assessment by comparing the fits of competing models – see later. The null deviance is given as 560 on 19 degrees of freedom; this is the value for a model including only an intercept. In fact, for the multiple linear regression model with a Gaussian error distribution, the deviance is more familiar as a *residual sum of squares*, and so the residual deviance of 2.156 on 13 degrees of freedom is simply the residual sum of squares after including the six explanatory variables in the model. The difference between the null deviance and the residual deviance, that is, the value 557.84, is the sum of squares due to regression on the six explanatory variables.

Usually in GLMs the difference in deviance for two *nested* models (one model contains terms that are additional to those in the other), can be tested approximately as a chi-square with degrees of freedom equal to the difference in the degrees of freedom of the two models. For the normal distribution, however, this approximate result need not be used since exact results are available; in this case since deviances are residual sums of squares, the difference in deviances can be related to the usual F statistic for testing the hypothesis that the regression coefficients are zero. This test involves a comparison of the mean square due to regression with the mean square about regression, that is, the term that estimates σ^2. In Table 1.2 the latter is simply what is called the *dispersion parameter* for the Gaussian family, 0.1658. (More will be said about dispersion parameters in Section 1.5). So we can now construct the familiar analysis of variance table for testing the hypothesis that the regression coefficients of all six explanatory variables are zero:

Analysis of variance table for multiple regression of hypertension data

Source	df	SS	MS	F
Due to regression	6	557.84	92.97	546.88
Residual	13	2.16	0.17	
Total	19	560.00		

The F-value is enormous and the associated p-value is tiny. Clearly the hypothesis that all six regression coefficients are zero can be rejected. Deciding whether some of the coefficients are zero and finding a more parsimonious model for the data are left as exercises for the reader (see Exercise 1.1).

As well as using the deviance, the quality of fit of a model should be assessed by examination of *residuals* and/or other *regression diagnostics*. Again for the (hopefully) more familiar multiple regression model this is left as an exercise for the reader (see Exercise 1.2).

1.3.2   Nodal involvement in prostatic cancer patients

The data shown in Table 1.3 arise from a study reported by Brown (1980) involving patients with cancer of the prostate. The aim was to determine whether a combination of five variables could be used to forecast whether or not the cancer has spread to the lymph nodes, since this forms the basis for the treatment regime that should be adopted. The 53 patients in the study had undergone a laparotomy to determine nodal involvement or not in their case. Here, then, the response variable (*nodal*) is binary with zero signifying the absence of and unity the presence of nodal involvement. Details of the explanatory variables are as follows:

x_1:   age of patient at diagnosis (years) – *age*
x_2:   level of serum acid phosphatase (in King–Armstrong units) – *acid*
x_3:   the result of an X-ray examination (0 = negative, 1 = positive) – *X-ray*
x_4:   the size of the tumour as determined by a rectal examination (0 = small, 1 = large) – *size*
x_5:   a summary of the pathological grade of the tumour determined from a biopsy (0 = less serious, 1 = more serious) – *grade*

Table 1.3 Data on patients with cancer of the prostate

	Age	*Acid*	*X-ray*	*Size*	*Grade*	*Nodal*
1	66	0.48	0	0	0	0
2	68	0.56	0	0	0	0
3	66	0.50	0	0	0	0
4	56	0.52	0	0	0	0
5	58	0.50	0	0	0	0
6	60	0.49	0	0	0	0
7	65	0.46	1	0	0	0
8	60	0.62	1	0	0	0
9	50	0.56	0	0	1	1
10	49	0.55	1	0	0	0
11	61	0.62	0	0	0	0
12	58	0.71	0	0	0	0
13	51	0.65	0	0	0	0
14	67	0.67	1	0	1	0
15	67	0.47	0	0	1	0
16	51	0.49	0	0	0	0
17	56	0.50	0	0	1	0
18	60	0.78	0	0	0	0
19	52	0.83	0	0	0	0
20	56	0.98	0	0	0	0
21	67	0.52	0	0	0	0
22	63	0.75	0	0	0	0
23	59	0.99	0	0	1	1
24	64	1.87	0	0	0	0
25	61	1.36	1	0	0	1
26	56	0.82	0	0	0	1
27	64	0.40	0	1	1	0
28	61	0.50	0	1	0	0
29	64	0.50	0	1	1	0
30	63	0.40	0	1	0	0
31	52	0.55	0	1	1	0
32	66	0.59	0	1	1	0
33	58	0.48	1	1	0	1
34	57	0.51	1	1	1	1
35	65	0.49	0	1	0	1
36	65	0.48	0	1	1	0
37	59	0.63	1	1	1	0
38	61	1.02	0	1	0	0
39	53	0.76	0	1	0	0
40	67	0.95	0	1	0	0
41	53	0.66	0	1	1	0
42	65	0.84	1	1	1	1
43	50	0.81	1	1	1	1
44	60	0.76	1	1	1	1
45	45	0.70	0	1	1	1
46	56	0.78	1	1	1	1
47	46	0.70	0	1	0	1
48	67	0.67	0	1	0	1
49	63	0.82	0	1	0	1
50	57	0.67	0	1	1	1
51	51	0.72	1	1	0	1
52	64	0.89	1	1	0	1
53	68	1.26	1	1	1	1

Source: Brown (1980).

Since the response variable is binary, we will fit a logistic regression model within the GLM framework. To begin, we shall consider the single explanatory variable, *age*. The estimated regression coefficient for age is -0.067, with an estimated standard error of 0.048. Interpretation of the regression coefficients in a logistic regression is as conditional log odds ratios (at least when there is more than a single explanatory variable, and when no interaction terms are present in the model). Interpretation becomes more straightforward if the coefficients are exponentiated so that they become conditional odds ratios. For age this leads to a value of 0.935; our fitted model has estimated that the odds of nodal involvement for patients aged $x + 1$ years is 0.935 times that of patients aged x years. It may be more practically useful to give the estimated odds ratio for, say, a five-year rather than a one-year difference; this is simply $\exp[5 \times (-0.067)] = 0.715$.

Of course, these point estimates are not very useful on their own; we need to construct an appropriate confidence interval. For a one-year age difference, the 95% confidence interval for the odds ratio is $[\exp(-0.067 - 1.96 \times 0.048), \exp(-0.067 + 1.96 \times 0.048)]$, giving the interval $[0.851, 1.027]$. The corresponding interval for a five-year age interval is $[\exp(5 \times (-0.067) - 1.96 \times 5 \times 0.048), \exp(5 \times (-0.067) + 1.96 \times 5 \times 0.048)]$, giving the interval $[0.447, 1.145]$. Since both intervals contain the value one, there is no evidence that age is predictive of the probability of nodal involvement.

Now let us look at the two explanatory variables, *age* and *acid*. The estimated regression coefficients and their standard errors are now:

	Estimated coefficient	Standard error
Age	−0.077	0.050
Acid	2.256	1.261

The fitted model is

$$\text{logit}\{\Pr(\text{nodal involvement})|\text{age, acid}\} = 2.349 - 0.077 \times \text{age} + 2.256 \times \text{acid} \tag{1.6}$$

so that the predicted probability of nodal involvement given age and acid is

$$\Pr(\text{nodal involvement}|\text{age, acid}) = \frac{\exp[2.349 - 0.077 \times \text{age} + 2.256 \times \text{acid}]}{1 + \exp[2.349 - 0.077 \times \text{age} + 0.256 \times \text{acid}]} \tag{1.7}$$

A plot of the predicted probabilities is shown in Figure 1.3, and in Figure 1.4 a 'smooth' fitted surface has been added to the diagram (see Chapter 4).

The results of fitting a logistic regression model which includes all five explanatory variables is shown in Table 1.4. (The estimated regression coefficients in the fitted model given in Table 1.4 correspond to the described 0/1 coding for the binary explanatory variables given above. In some software packages such two-category explanatory variables are automatically recoded as $1/-1$, in which case the estimated regression coefficients and their standard errors will need to be doubled to give the values in Table 1.4.) The regression coefficient for size of tumour, for example, is estimated to be 2.04, with a standard error of 0.82; the corresponding estimated odds ratio is $\exp(2.04) = 7.69$, and the approximate 95% confidence interval is given by $[\exp(2.04 - 1.96 \times 0.82), \exp(2.04 + 1.96 \times 0.82)]$ or $[1.54, 38.37]$. Consequently,

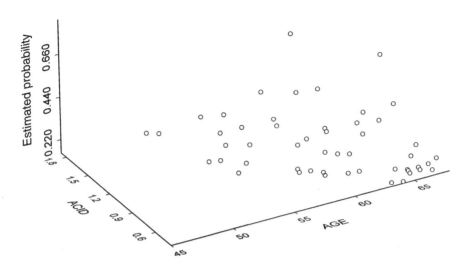

Figure 1.3   Estimated probability of nodal involvement from a logistic regression model fitted to prostate cancer data using age and acid as exploratory variables.

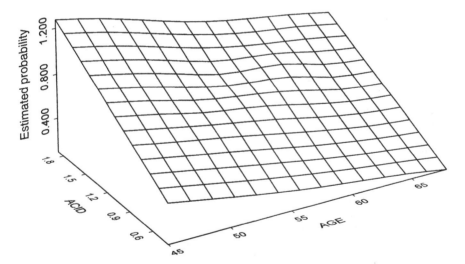

Figure 1.4   Estimated probability of nodal involvement from a logistic regression model fitted to prostate cancer data using age and acid as exploratory variables, with fitted surface.

conditional on the values of the other four explanatory variables remaining the same, for a large tumour the odds ratio of the presence of nodal involvement to the absence of nodal involvement is between one and a half and nearly 40 times as large as for a small tumour. The width of the confidence interval is, however, rather disturbing, and

Table 1.4   Results from a logistic regression model fitted to the cancer data in Table 1.3

Covariates	Estimated regression coefficient	Standard error	Estimate/SE
Intercept	1.517	3.554	0.427
Age	−0.099	0.061	−1.619
Acid	2.638	1.323	1.993
X-ray	1.683	0.799	2.107
Size	2.040	0.823	2.480
Grade	0.345	0.795	0.435

(Dispersion parameter for binomial family taken to be 1.)
Null deviance: 69.17 on 52 degrees of freedom.
Residual deviance: 46.69 on 47 degrees of freedom.

Table 1.5   Comparison of logistic regression models for the prostate cancer example

Explanatory variables included	Deviance	df	Change in deviance	Change in df
None	69.17	52	–	–
Size	59.42	51	9.69	1
Size, X-ray	52.99	50	6.43	1
Size, X-ray, acid	49.81	49	3.18	1
Size, X-ray, acid, age	46.88	48	2.93	1
Size, X-ray, acid, age, grade	46.69	47	0.19	1

in practice it would certainly be necessary to investigate the possibility of interactions between factors and perhaps to consider transforming some of the explanatory variables (see Exercise 1.3).

To compare two nested models for binomial data (the generally assumed distribution when using logistic regression), no exact distribution theory is available for differences in deviance values. But, as mentioned previously, as an approximation, the difference can be judged as a chi-square with degrees of freedom equal to the difference in the degrees of freedom of the competing models. For example, in Table 1.4 the difference in the null deviance and the residual deviance has the value 22.48, and the corresponding difference in degrees of freedom is 5. (The difference in deviance is simply the likelihood ratio test.) Using the chi-square distribution the associated p-value is less than 0.001, so we can clearly claim that some of the five variables at least make a contribution to the prediction of nodal involvement. Let us see if we can say a little more here by considering adding the variables to the null model in an order suggested by the absolute values of the ratios of the estimated regression coefficients to their standard errors in Table 1.4 and comparing the corresponding deviances. The results are shown in Table 1.5. It appears that only the size of the tumour and the result of an X-ray are important in predicting nodal involvement.

1.3.3   Byssinosis and dust in the workplace

The data shown in Table 1.6 come from a survey of workers in the US cotton industry, and record whether they were suffering from byssinosis, as well as the values of five explanatory variables: the race of the worker, the sex of the worker, the smoking

Table 1.6   Dustiness in the work place (Taken with permission of the International Statistical Institute from Higgins and Koch, 1977.)

Presence of byssinosis		Dust	Race	Sex	Smoking	EmpLength
Yes	*No*					
3	37	1	1	1	1	1
0	74	2	1	1	1	1
2	258	3	1	1	1	1
25	139	1	2	1	1	1
0	88	2	2	1	1	1
3	242	3	2	1	1	1
0	5	1	1	2	1	1
1	93	2	1	2	1	1
3	180	3	1	2	1	1
2	22	1	2	2	1	1
2	145	2	2	2	1	1
3	260	3	2	2	1	1
0	16	1	1	1	2	1
0	35	2	1	1	2	1
0	134	3	1	1	2	1
6	75	1	2	1	2	1
1	47	2	2	1	2	1
1	122	3	2	1	2	1
0	4	1	1	2	2	1
1	54	2	1	2	2	1
2	169	3	1	2	2	1
1	24	1	2	2	2	1
3	142	2	2	2	2	1
4	301	3	2	2	2	1
8	21	1	1	1	1	2
1	50	2	1	1	1	2
1	187	3	1	1	1	2
8	30	1	2	1	1	2
0	5	2	2	1	1	2
0	33	3	2	1	1	2
0	0	1	1	2	1	2
1	33	2	1	2	1	2
2	94	3	1	2	1	2
0	0	1	2	2	1	2
0	4	2	2	2	1	2
0	3	3	2	2	1	2
2	8	1	1	1	2	2
1	16	2	1	1	2	2
0	58	3	1	1	2	2
1	9	1	2	1	2	2
0	0	2	2	1	2	2
0	7	3	2	1	2	2
0	0	1	1	2	2	2
0	30	2	1	2	2	2
1	90	3	1	2	2	2
0	0	1	2	2	2	2
0	4	2	2	2	2	2
0	4	3	2	2	2	2
31	77	1	1	1	1	3
1	141	2	1	1	1	3
12	495	3	1	1	1	3

(*Continued*)

Table 1.6   *(Continued)*

Presence of byssinosis		Dust	Race	Sex	Smoking	EmpLength
Yes	No					
10	31	1	2	1	1	3
0	1	2	2	1	1	3
0	45	3	2	1	1	3
0	1	1	1	2	1	3
3	91	2	1	2	1	3
3	176	3	1	2	1	3
0	1	1	2	2	1	3
0	0	2	2	2	1	3
0	2	3	2	2	1	3
5	47	1	1	1	2	3
0	39	2	1	1	2	3
3	182	3	1	1	2	3
3	15	1	2	1	2	3
0	1	2	2	1	2	3
0	23	3	2	1	2	3
0	2	1	1	2	2	3
3	187	2	1	2	2	3
2	340	3	1	2	2	3
0	0	1	2	2	2	3
0	2	2	2	2	2	3
0	3	3	2	2	2	3

Dust:	dustiness of workplace (1 = high, 2 = medium, 3 = low).
Race:	ethnic group of worker (1 = white, 2 = other).
Sex:	1 = male, 2 = female.
Smoking:	smoking status (1 = smoker, 2 = non-smoker).
EmpLength:	length of employment (1 = less than 10 years, 2 = 10–20 years, 3 = over 20 years).

status of the worker, the length of the worker's employment and the dustiness of the workplace. Interest lies in determining how the explanatory variables are related to the presence of byssinosis, in particular how the condition is related to the dustiness of the workplace. Here the original binary responses relating to the presence or absence of the condition have been grouped for all workers with the same values of the five explanatory variables.

Once again logistic regression can be used to investigate these data, and the results of applying the logistic regression model to the data in Table 1.6, including all explanatory variables, are shown in Table 1.7. Note that several observations are not used in the analysis; these observations correspond to combinations of values of the explanatory variables that were not observed in any worker.

In this analysis dustiness of the workplace and employment length have been used as quasi-continuous variables with the values 1, 2 and 3, rather than being recoded in terms of two dummy variables each. The latter possibility is left as an exercise for the reader (see Exercise 1.4). It appears that dustiness is of overwhelming importance in predicting the presence of byssinosis in a worker, with smoking and employment length also of some importance. This is confirmed if we compare the deviances of a model including only dustiness, smoking and employment and a model including all five explanatory variables. These values turn out to be 73 (61 df) and 70 (59 df). The difference of 3 with 2 degrees of freedom is not significant when judged as a

Table 1.7 Results of fitting a logistic regression model to the data in Table 1.6

Covariates	Estimated regression coefficient	Standard error	Estimate/SE
(Intercept)	−0.485	0.606	−0.801
Race	0.246	0.206	1.195
Sex	−0.259	0.212	−1.224
Smoking	−0.629	0.193	−3.259
Dust	−1.375	0.115	−11.902
Emp	0.386	0.107	3.607

(Dispersion parameter for binomial family taken to be 1.)
Null deviance: 322.53 on 64 degrees of freedom.
Residual deviance: 69.51 on 59 degrees of freedom.
7 observations deleted due to missing values.

chi-square; consequently, race and sex do not appear of importance in predicting the occurrence of byssinosis.

A range of residuals and other diagnostics are available for use in association with logistic regression to check whether particular components of the model are adequate. A comprehensive account of these is given in Collett (1991). Here we shall demonstrate only the use of what is known as the *deviance residual*; this is the signed square root of the contribution of the ith observation to the overall deviance. Explicitly, it is given by

$$d_i = \text{sgn}(y_i - \hat{y}_i) \left[2y_i \log\left(\frac{y_i}{\hat{y}_i}\right) + 2(n_i - y_i)\log\left(\frac{n_i - y_i}{n_i - \hat{y}_i}\right) \right]^{1/2} \qquad (1.8)$$

where y_i is the observed number of 'successes' for the ith observation (the number of people with byssinosis for each combination of covariates in our example), and $\hat{y}_i$ is its predicted value from the fitted model; $\text{sgn}(y_i - \hat{y}_i)$ is the function that makes d_i positive when $y_i \geq \hat{y}_i$ and negative when $y_i < \hat{y}_i$. The residual provides information about how well the model fits each particular observation.

In Figure 1.5, deviance residuals are plotted against the fitted values and largely fall into a horizontal band between −2 and 2. This pattern does not suggest a poor fit for any particular observation or subset of observations.

1.4 Poisson regression

Multiple regression and logistic regression will almost certainly be familiar to most readers, and the previous section has been largely an exercise in describing how both types of model are applied via the generalized estimation framework. But readers may be less familiar with another form of regression model that is also subsumed under the GLM heading, namely *Poisson regression*. The Poisson regression model is useful for response variables that are counts or frequencies and for which it is reasonable to assume an underlying *Poisson distribution*, that is, the distribution

$$\Pr(y) = \frac{\mu^y e^{-\mu}}{y!}, \qquad y = 0, 1, 2, \ldots \qquad (1.9)$$

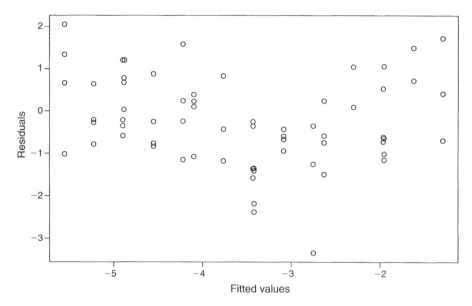

Figure 1.5   Plot of deviance residuals from logistic regression model fitted to the byssinosis data.

For exploring the relationship between the mean of a Poisson variable and some explanatory variables of interest, the link function in a GLM is generally taken to be the logarithm, guaranteeing positive fitted values, although the identity link is also occasionally used. We will now examine some examples of the application of this form of regression.

1.4.1   Remembering stressful events

The data shown in Table 1.8 are given by Haberman (1978), and also by Seeber (1998). They arise from asking randomly chosen household members from a probability sample of a town in the USA which stressful events had occurred within the last 18 months and to report the month of occurrence of these events. A scattergram of the data (see Figure 1.6) indicates a decline in the number of events as these lay further in the past, the result perhaps of the fallibility of human memory.

Since the response variable here is a count, we shall use Poisson regression to investigate the relationship of recalls with time; explicitly, the model to be fitted to the mean number of recalls, μ, is

$$\log(\mu) = \beta_0 + \beta_1 \times \text{time} \tag{1.10}$$

The results of the fitting procedure are shown in Table 1.9. The estimated regression coefficient for time is -0.084 with an estimated standard error of 0.017. Exponentiating equation (1.10) and inserting the estimated parameter values gives

$$\hat{\mu} = 16.5 \times 0.920^{\text{time}} \tag{1.11}$$

The scattergram of the original data showing also the fitted model is given in Figure 1.7. The difference in deviance of the null model and one including time as an explanatory variable is large and clearly indicates that the regression coefficient for time is not zero.

Table 1.8   Distribution, by months prior to interview, of stressful events reported from subjects; 147 subjects reporting exactly one stressful event in the period from 1 to 18 months prior to interview

Time	1	2	3	4	5	6	7	8	9	10	11	12	13	14	15	16	17	18
y	15	11	14	17	5	11	10	4	8	10	7	9	11	3	6	1	1	4

Source: Haberman (1978), with permission.

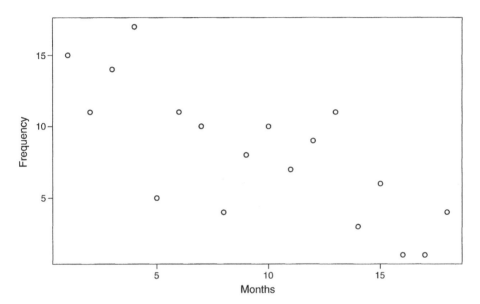

Figure 1.6   Scatterplot of remembering stressful events data.

Table 1.9   Results of a Poisson regression on the data in Table 1.8

Covariates	Estimated regression coefficient	Standard error	Estimate/SE
Intercept	2.803	0.148	18.920
Time	−0.084	0.017	−4.987

(Dispersion parameter for Poisson family taken to be 1.)
Null deviance: 50.84 on 17 degrees of freedom.
Residual deviance: 24.57 on 16 degrees of freedom.

1.4.2   Recurrences of superficial bladder cancer

The data in Table 1.10 were originally reported in Seeber (1989) and are also given in Seeber (1998). The data arise from 31 male patients who have been treated for superficial bladder cancer, and give the number of recurrent tumours during a particular time after removal of the primary tumour, and the size of the tumour (whether smaller or larger than 3 cm).

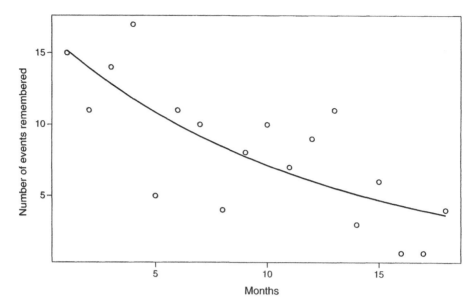

Figure 1.7 Scatterplot of remembering stressful events data, showing the fitted Poisson regression model.

Table 1.10 Bladder cancer data

Time	x	n	Time	x	n
2	0	1	13	0	2
3	0	1	15	0	2
6	0	1	18	0	2
8	0	1	23	0	2
9	0	1	20	0	3
10	0	1	24	0	4
11	0	1	1	1	1
13	0	1	5	1	1
14	0	1	17	1	1
16	0	1	18	1	1
21	0	1	25	1	1
22	0	1	18	1	2
24	0	1	25	1	2
26	0	1	4	1	3
27	0	1	19	1	4
7	0	2			

$x = 0$, tumour < 3 cm; $x = 1$, tumour > 3 cm.
Source: Seeber (1998), taken with permission of the publishers, John Wiley and Sons, Ltd.

Before coming to the analysis of the data in Table 1.10, we first need to introduce the idea of a *Poisson process*, in which the waiting times between successive events of interest (the tumours in this case) are independent and exponentially distributed with common mean, $1/\lambda$. Then the number of events that occur up to time t has a Poisson distribution

Table 1.11 Results from fitting Poisson regression model to bladder cancer data

Covariates	Estimated regression coefficient	Standard error	Estimate/SE
Intercept	−2.339	0.177	−13.235
x	0.229	0.306	0.749

(Dispersion parameter for Poisson family taken to be 1.)
Null deviance: 25.96 on 30 degrees of freedom.
Residual deviance: 25.42 on 29 degrees of freedom.

with mean $\mu = \lambda t$. The parameter of interest is the rate at which events occur, and for a single explanatory variable, x, we can adopt a Poisson regression approach,

$$\log \lambda = \beta_0 + \beta_1 x \tag{1.12}$$

for modelling the dependence of λ on x. This model can be rewritten in terms of μ as

$$\log \mu = \beta_0 + \beta_1 x + \log t \tag{1.13}$$

In this model $\log t$ is a variable in the model whose regression coefficient is fixed at unity; this is usually known as an *offset*.

For the data in Table 1.10 we wish to apply the model in (1.13), with x being a binary variable labelling size of tumour, $x = 1$ for those above 3 cm and $x = 0$ otherwise. The results of fitting the Poisson regression model in this case are shown in Table 1.11. Exponentiating the model for $\log \lambda$ in (1.12) gives

$$\lambda = e^{\beta_0} \left(e^{\beta_1} \right)^x \tag{1.14}$$

So for smaller tumours, where $x = 0$, the estimate of λ is $\exp(-2.34) = 0.096$; for larger tumours it is $\exp(0.229) = 1.26$ times as large. (Confidence intervals can be found in the usual way; see Exercise 1.5.) In terms of waiting times between recurrences, the mean for smaller tumours is estimated to be $1/0.096 = 10.4$ months, and for larger tumours $1/(1.26 \times 0.096) = 8.3$ months.

1.5 Overdispersion

An important aspect of GLMs that thus far we have largely ignored is the variance function, $V(\mu)$, which captures how the variance of a response variable depends upon its mean. The general form of the relationship is

$$\text{Var(response)} = \phi V(\mu) \tag{1.15}$$

where ϕ is a constant and $V(\mu)$ specifies how the variance depends on the mean μ. For the error distributions considered previously this general form becomes:

Normal: $V(\mu) = 1$, $\phi = \sigma^2$; here the variance does not depend on the mean.
Binomial: $V(\mu) = \mu(1 - \mu)$, $\phi = 1$.
Poisson: $V(\mu) = \mu$, $\phi = 1$.

In the case of a Poisson variable we see that the mean and variance are equal, and in the case of a binomial variable where the mean is the probability of the occurrence of the event of interest, p, the variance is $p(1 - p)$.

Both the Poisson and binomial distributions have variance functions that are completely determined by the mean. There is no free parameter for the variance since in applications of the GLM with binomial or Poisson error distributions the dispersion parameter, ϕ, is defined to be 1 (see previous results for logistic and Poisson regression). But in some applications this becomes too restrictive to fully account for the empirical variance in the data; in such cases it is common to describe the phenomenon as *overdispersion*. For example, if the response variable is the proportion of family members who have been ill in the past year, observed in a large number of families, then the individual binary observations that make up the observed proportions are likely to be correlated rather than independent. This non-independence can lead to a variance that is greater (less) than that on the assumption of binomial variability. And observed counts often exhibit larger variance than would be expected from the Poisson assumption, a fact noted over 80 years ago by Greenwood and Yule (1920). Greenwood and Yule's suggested solution to the problem was a model in which μ was a random variable with a gamma distribution, leading to a *negative binomial distribution* for the count.

There are a number of strategies for accommodating overdispersion, but here we concentrate on a relatively simple approach which retains the use of the binomial or Poisson error distributions as appropriate, but allows estimation of a value of ϕ from the data rather than defining it to be unity for these distributions. The estimate is usually the residual deviance divided by its degrees of freedom, exactly the method used with Gaussian models. Parameter estimates remain the same but parameter standard errors are increased by multiplying them by the square root of the estimated dispersion parameter. This process can be carried out manually; (almost) equivalently, the overdispersed model can be formally fitted using a procedure known as *quasi-likelihood*; this allows estimation of model parameters without fully knowing the error distribution of the response variable – see McCullagh and Nelder (1989) for full technical details of the approach.

When fitting GLMs with binomial or Poisson error distributions, overdispersion can often be spotted by comparing the residual deviance with its degrees of freedom. For a well-fitting model the two quantities should be approximately equal. If the deviance is far greater than the degrees of freedom overdispersion may be indicated. An example will help to clarify these points.

1.5.1 Colonic polyps

Giardiello *et al.* (1993) and Piantadosi (1997) give data from a placebo-controlled trial of a non-steroidal anti-inflammatory drug in the treatment of familial adenomatous polyposis (FAP). The trial was halted after a planned interim analysis had suggested compelling evidence in favour of the treatment. The response variable in this case was the number of colonic polyps at 12 months. A data set based on the results from this study is shown in Table 1.12.

The results of fitting a Poisson regression model to these data, using treatment coded as a 0/1 dummy variable and age as covariates, are shown in Table 1.13. The residual deviance is about ten times its degrees of freedom, a clear sign of overdispersion. Refitting the model using the quasi-likelihood approach to force the estimation of the dispersion parameter gives the results shown in Table 1.14. (The estimated dispersion parameter is very similar to the values obtained from Table 1.13 by dividing the residual deviance by its degrees of freedom, that is, $179.5/17 = 10.56$.)

Table 1.12 Colonic polyps data

Number	63	2	28	17	61	1	7	15	44	25	3	28	10	40	33	46	50	3	1	4
Treat	0	1	0	1	0	1	0	0	0	1	1	0	0	0	1	0	0	1	1	1
Age	20	16	18	22	13	23	34	50	19	17	23	22	30	27	23	22	34	23	22	42

Source: Piantadosi (1997), taken with permission of the publisher, John Wiley and Sons, Ltd.

Table 1.13 Poisson regression results for colonic polyps data

Covariates	Estimated regression coefficient	Standard error	Estimate/SE
Intercept	4.529	0.147	30.851
Treat	−1.359	0.117	−11.594
Age	−0.039	0.006	−6.524

(Dispersion parameter for Poisson family taken to be 1.)
Null deviance: 378.66 on 19 degrees of freedom.
Residual deviance: 179.54 on 17 degrees of freedom.

Table 1.14 Results from fitting a Poisson regression model to the colonic polyps data, allowing for overdispersion

Covariates	Estimated regression coefficient	Standard error	Estimate/SE
Intercept	4.529	0.479	9.445
Treat	−1.359	0.382	−3.549
Age	−0.039	0.020	−1.997

(Dispersion parameter for quasi-likelihood family taken to be 10.56.)
Null deviance: 378.66 on 19 degrees of freedom.
Residual deviance: 179.54 on 17 degrees of freedom.
Number of Fisher scoring iterations: 4.

The estimated dispersion parameter is now used to adjust the standard errors of the regression coefficients of age and treatment, giving $0.117 \times \sqrt{10.56} = 0.382$ for the latter and $0.006 \times \sqrt{10.56} = 0.020$ for the former. The z-values associated with each variable are now considerably reduced in value compared to those given in Table 1.13. But treatment remains highly significant, with age becoming less so. Looking at deviance values for models including only age and then age and treatment, however, leads to the conclusion that age does need to be included. (The deviance values are 228.6 with 18 df and 179.5 with 17 df.)

A possible reason for the occurrence of overdispersion in these data is that polyps do not occur independently of one another, and may 'cluster' together. If so, it would lead to the extra variation observed.

A full discussion of overdispersion is given in Collett (1991) and in McCullagh and Nelder (1989).

1.6   Summary

Generalized linear models provide a very powerful and flexible framework for the application of regression models to medical data. Some familiarity with the basis of such models might allow medical researchers to consider more realistic models for their data, rather than to rely solely on linear and logistic regression.

Software

All major software packages contain a component for fitting generalized linear models. Usage is generally very straightforward, the user needing simply to identify the particular data set to be analysed, select the response and explanatory variables, and finally choose the relevant link function and error distributions. In most cases, the identity link and Gaussian errors are the defaults.

The generalized linear model procedures in three major packages are:

SAS   `proc genmod`
STATA   `glm command`
S-PLUS   `glm function`

Further information about these packages can be obtained from the following websites:

SAS   http://www.sas.com
STATA   http://www.stata.com
S-PLUS   http://www.splus.com

Detailed code for fitting GLMs using each of these packages is available in Der and Everitt (2001), Rabe-Hesketh and Everitt (2000) and Everitt (2001b).

Exercises

1.1 Investigate the hypertension data in Table 1.1, to try to find the most parsimonious model that adequately describes the observations.

1.2 Having decided upon a suitable model for the hypertension data, examine some suitable plots of the various residuals and other regression diagnostics available in the statistical software package you are using.

1.3 In his analysis of the prostatic cancer data in Table 1.3, Collett (1991) suggests using $\log(acid)$ rather than $acid$ as an explanatory variable, since the distribution of values of the original variable is rather skew. Investigate this possibility and that of including interactions between, in particular, *size* and *grade*, and *grade* and $\log(acid)$, in the model.

1.4 Rerun the logistic regression on the byssinosis data in Table 1.6, now recoding both dustiness of the workplace and employment length as suitable dummy variables. What difference does this make to the conclusions of the analysis?

1.5 For the data in Table 1.9 find a 95% confidence interval for the rate of occurrence of recurrent tumours in the group of patients whose primary tumour was larger than 3 cm.

2
Generalized Linear Models for Longitudinal Data

2.1 Introduction

Generalized linear models have, as described in the previous chapter, unified regression analysis for discrete and continuous response variables in situations where there is a single measurement of the response on each individual in the study. But medical investigations, particularly those that involve the assessment of competing treatments, for example, *clinical trials*, rarely result in a one-time final result for a patient. Generally clinicians wish to follow the evolution of a patient's health over a period of time. Consequently, in the majority of clinical trials and in other types of study, the primary outcome variable is observed on several occasions throughout the investigation. Such *longitudinal studies* have become increasingly popular in medicine, where they have proven to be of importance for understanding the development and persistence of disease and for identifying factors that can alter the course of disease development. For example, in studies such as the Framingham Heart Study (Dawber, 1980) and the Six Cities Study of Air Pollution and Health (Ware *et al.*, 1984; Dockery *et al.*, 1989), investigators have followed populations of different ages over time to study the development of chronic illnesses and to detect risk factors for disease. And the majority of clinical trials provide a rich source of longitudinal data, as we shall see in the examples to be used in this chapter.

The distinguishing feature of a longitudinal study is that the response variable of interest and a set of explanatory variables (covariates) are measured repeatedly over time. The main objective in such a study is to characterize change in the response variable over time and to determine the covariates most associated with any change. Because observations of the response variable are made on the same individual at different times, it is likely that the repeated responses for the same person will be correlated with each other. This correlation must be taken into account to draw valid and efficient inferences about parameters of scientific interest. It is the likely presence of such correlation that makes modelling longitudinal data more complex than dealing with a single response value for each individual; this is particularly so in the case of repeated non-normal responses, for example, binary responses, where different assumptions about the source of the correlation can lead to regression coefficients with distinct interpretations.

2.2   Marginal and conditional regression models

With a single value of the response variable available for each subject, modelling is restricted to the expected or average value of the response among persons with the same values of the covariates. But with repeated observations on each individual, there are other possibilities, which may be of importance in particular circumstances. We need to distinguish between longitudinal studies where the *marginal expectation* of the responses is of scientific interest and studies where the *conditional expectation* of the responses is of more relevance.

2.2.1   Marginal models

Marginal models for longitudinal studies are the direct analogues, for the repeated measures encountered in such studies, of the generalized linear model described in Chapter 1. With such models interest focuses on the regression parameters of each response separately, sometimes referred to as the *cross-sectional mean response*. We model the relationship of this marginal mean and the explanatory variables separately from the within-subject correlation. The term 'marginal' implies that we are concerned with each response separately, conditional on the covariates, but not on the other responses. The essentials of the generalized model for this situation look very similar to those given in Section 1.2 for a single response:

$$g(\mu_j) = \beta_0 + \beta_1 x_{1j} + \beta_2 x_{2j} + \cdots + \beta_q x_{qj} \tag{2.1}$$

$$V_j = \phi V(\mu_j) \tag{2.2}$$

where now μ_j is the expected value of the response and $x_{1j}, x_{2j}, ..., x_{qj}$ are the values of the q covariates when measured on the jth occasion. For simplicity of description we shall assume that each individual has T repeated measures of the response, although this is not an essential requirement; it is relatively straightforward to deal both with differing numbers of repeated measures and differing times at which the measures are taken for each individual. As formulated in (2.1), the model allows for covariates which have different values on each occasion the response is measured; however, for some covariates, for example, treatment group in a clinical trial, the value will remain constant over time. For this type of model the regression coefficients have the same interpretation as in the case of a GLM for a single response, as we shall illustrate later.

The additional component needed in the model specified in (2.1) and (2.2) to make it suitable for longitudinal data is one that allows for the possibility that the repeated responses may be correlated. In practice, this involves choosing one of a number of potentially useful functions for modelling the correlations in terms of a (hopefully) small number of additional parameters, say, $\theta_1, \theta_2, ..., \theta_m$. Formally, this component of the model is represented as follows:

$$\text{corr}(y_j, y_k) = f(\mu_i, \mu_k; \boldsymbol{\theta}) \tag{2.3}$$

where f is a known function, $\boldsymbol{\theta}' = [\theta_1, \theta_2, ..., \theta_m]$ (the prime indicating matrix or vector transposition) and y_j and y_k are the responses on occasions j and k. (This part of the modelling process will become clearer when we come to describe some specific examples.)

Although the GLM for the single-response situation is easily extended in principle to the repeated-response situation that occurs in a longitudinal study, a complication arises when it comes to actually estimating the parameters of the new model. For other than Gaussian models with an identity link function, the likelihood is often intractable because of the presence of many *nuisance* parameters, in addition to the parameters of primary concern (the βs and the θs). The reasons why this is so are set out in detail in Diggle *et al.* (1994) and need not concern us here. Our interest lies more in what can be done to deal with the problem in practice. There are two distinct possibilities.

One approach is to assume the repeated responses are independent of one another – the *independence working model*. Standard GLM software can now be used for estimation after the data has been reorganized (if necessary) so that each individual contributes as many records as they have repeated measures (see later for examples). A question that needs to be addressed if this approach is contemplated is how wrong it is likely to be when the repeated measures on the same individual are correlated. It can be shown that the approach will still give *consistent* estimates of the regression parameters, that is, with large samples, the point estimates should be close to the true population values. Unfortunately, however, assuming independence is likely to lead to standard errors that are too small for between-subjects covariates (assuming the correlation within individuals is positive), since they are based on the belief that we have more independent data points than is really the case.

The next question might be whether there is anything that can be done to 'fix-up' these standard errors so that we can still apply standard GLM software to get reasonably satisfactory results on longitudinal data. Two approaches which can often help to obtain more suitable estimates of the required standard errors are *bootstrapping* and use of the *robust variance estimator* (also known as the *sandwich* or *Huber–White* variance estimator).

The idea underlying the bootstrap, a technique described in detail in Efron and Tibshirani (1993), is to resample from the observed data with replacement to achieve a sample of the same size each time, and to use the variation in the estimated parameters across the set of bootstrap samples in order to obtain a value for the sampling variability of the estimates. With correlated data, the bootstrap sample needs to be drawn with replacement from the set of independent subjects, so that intra-subject correlation is preserved in the bootstrap samples (more details later).

The sandwich estimate of variance (see Everitt and Pickles, 2000, for complete details, including an explicit definition), involves, unlike the bootstrap which is computationally intensive, a closed-form calculation based on an asymptotic (large-sample) approximation; it is known to provide good results in many situations.

An alternative to assuming the independence of the repeated measurements is to use a method that fully utilizes information on the data's structure, including dependencies over time. This would lead to more efficient parameter estimates, that is, ones with lower variance. Maximizing the likelihood would be (asymptotically) the most efficient such method, but, as mentioned above, it is only a practical possibility for Gaussian responses, as described in detail in Everitt and Pickles (2000). In other cases there is often no suitable likelihood function with a required combination of the link, error distribution and correlation structure. To overcome the problem, Liang and Zeger (1986) and Zeger and Liang (1986) introduced a general method for incorporating within-subject correlation in GLMs, which is essentially an extension of the quasilikelihood approach mentioned briefly in the previous chapter; it is known as the *generalized estimating equation* (GEE) approach. (For an identity link function and Gaussian errors, the GEE approach is essentially equivalent to maximum likelihood estimation.)

The primary idea behind the GEE approach is that since the parameters specifying the structure of the correlation matrix are rarely of great practical interest, simple structures are used for the within-subject correlations, giving rise to the so-called *working correlation matrix*. Liang and Zeger (1986) show that the estimates of the parameters of most interest, that is, those that determine the average responses over time, are still valid even when the correlation structure is incorrectly specified, although their standard errors might remain poorly estimated if the working correlation matrix is far from the truth. But as with the independence situation described previously, this potential difficulty can often be handled satisfactorily by again using the sandwich estimator to find more reasonable standard errors. Possibilities for the working correlation matrix that are most frequently used in practice are as follows:

- An identity matrix, corresponding to the independence working model described above. Repeated responses are naïvely assumed to be independent, and standard generalized linear modelling software can be used for estimation etc., with each individual contributing as many records as repeated measures. Although clearly not realistic for most situations, used in association with a sandwich estimator of standard errors, it can lead to sensible inferences and has the distinct advantage of being simple to implement.

- An *exchangeable correlation matrix* with a single parameter, θ, which gives the correlation of each pair of repeated measures. This assumption leads to the so called *compound symmetry* structure for the covariance matrix of these measures, which may be familiar to many readers from their knowledge of repeated measures analysis of variance (Everitt, 2001a). If not, compound symmetry is explained in more detail in Section 2.2.2.

- An *autoregressive correlation matrix* also with a single parameter, but in which $\text{corr}(y_j,y_k) = \theta^{|k-j|}$, $j \neq k$. With $\theta < 1$ this gives a pattern in which repeated measures further apart in time are less correlated than those that are closer to one another.

- An unstructured correlation matrix with $T(T-1)/2$ parameters in which $\text{corr}(y_j,y_k) = \theta_{jk}$. In general, using this form is not attractive because of the excess of parameters involved.

In cases of possible overdispersion, the scale parameter, ϕ, in (2.2) can again be estimated as outlined in Chapter 1.

2.2.2   Conditional regression models

Marginal regression models as described in the previous subsection represent an intuitively recognizable extension of the model described in Chapter 1. But in longitudinal studies it may also be of interest to consider the conditional expectation of each response, given either the values of previous responses or a set of *random effects* that reflect natural heterogeneity amongst individuals due to unmeasured factors. In the case of the usual linear model with a Gaussian error model, Diggle *et al.* (1994) show that it is possible to formulate the different approaches so that the resulting regression coefficients have the same interpretation; but this is not the case with, for example, logistic regression, as we shall try to explain in what follows.

Random effects models

Random effects models formalize the sensible idea that an individual's pattern of responses in a study is likely to depend on many characteristics of that individual, including some that are unobserved. These unobserved characteristics are then included in the model as random variables, that is to say, random effects. The essential feature of a random effects model for longitudinal data is that there is natural heterogeneity across individuals in their regression coefficients and that this heterogeneity can be represented by an appropriate probability distribution. Correlation among observations from the same individual arises from them sharing unobserved variables, for example, a propensity to the illness under investigation, or a predisposition to exaggerate symptoms perhaps. Conditional on the values of these random effects, the repeated measurements of the response variable are assumed to be independent, the so-called *local independence assumption*. The aim now is to model the conditional mean (and variance) of the response on a particular occasion, given the random effects. The GLM in Chapter 1 needs to be amended as follows:

$$g(\mu_j^c) = \beta_0 + \beta_1 x_{1j} + \beta_2 x_{2j} + \cdots + \beta_q x_{qj} + u_1 z_{1j} + u_2 z_{2j} + \cdots + u_r z_{rj} \quad (2.4)$$

$$V_j^c = \phi V(\mu_j^c) \quad (2.5)$$

where μ_j^c is the conditional mean on occasion j, given the values of $u_1, u_2, \ldots, u_r$, terms that represent random variables having a multivariate normal distribution with mean vector the null vector, and an unknown covariance matrix, Σ; V_j^c is the conditional variance. The zs represent another set of explanatory variables (often, but not necessarily, a subset of the xs); see later for examples. Unlike the marginal models of the previous subsection, no correlation component is needed here, since the random effects themselves account directly for the correlations.

The random effects model specified in (2.4) becomes more transparent if we consider specific examples. Here we shall look at a simple situation in which, for a Gaussian response, there is, in addition to time, a single covariate, treatment group with two levels. To simplify the discussion we shall assume that there is no group × time interaction. We shall examine two models.

In the *random intercepts* model $r = 1$ and z_{1j} in (2.4) is equal to one. Since we are assuming a Gaussian response we will use an identity link function, and the model for y_{ij}, the response given by individual i at time t_j (or on occasion j), can be written explicitly as

$$y_{ij} = \beta_0 + \beta_1 \text{group}_i + \beta_2 t_j + u_i + \varepsilon_{ij} \quad (2.6)$$

with ε_{ij} having a normal distribution with mean zero and variance σ^2, and u_i having a normal distribution with mean zero and variance σ_u^2. (The ε_{ij} and u_i terms are assumed independent of one another.) Treatment group is indicated by the dummy variable 'group'.

In this case the random effect, u_i, models possible heterogeneity in the intercepts of the individuals, but each individual's trend over time is assumed parallel to their treatment group's average trend. The model is illustrated graphically in Figure 2.1.

The presence of the u_i terms in (2.6) implies that the repeated measurements of the response have what is known as a *compound symmetry pattern* for their covariance matrix; specifically, the diagonal elements are each given by $\sigma^2 + \sigma_u^2$, and the off-diagonal elements are each equal to σ_u^2.

In the *random intercepts and slopes* model $r = 2$ with z_{1j} and z_{2j} in (2.4) being equal to one and t_j respectively. The model is now given by;

$$y_{ij} = \beta_0 + \beta_1 \text{group}_i + \beta_2 t_j + u_{i1} + u_{i2} t_j + \varepsilon_{ij} \quad (2.7)$$

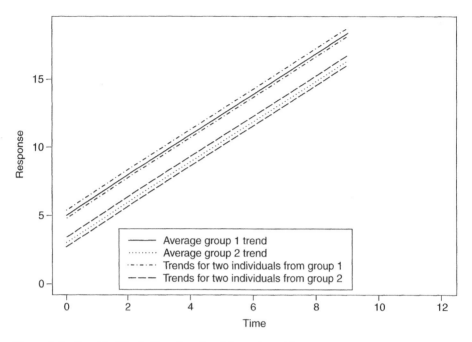

Figure 2.1   Graphical illustration of random intercept model.

Again the ε_{ij} are assumed normally distributed with zero mean and variance σ^2; the two random effects u_{i1} and u_{i2} are assumed to have a bivariate normal distribution with both means zero, variances $\sigma^2_{u_1}$ and $\sigma^2_{u_2}$, and covariance $\sigma_{u_1 u_2}$. (Again ε_{ij} is assumed independent of u_{i1} and u_{i2}.)

In this model, heterogeneity in both intercepts and slopes is modelled, with individuals deviating in terms of both slope and intercept from the average trend in their group. The model is illustrated graphically in Figure 2.2.

The presence of the two random effects, u_{i1} and u_{i2}, in (2.7) allows the covariance matrix of the repeated measurements of the response to have variances and covariances that change over time. Deriving the explicit form of the covariance matrix is left as an exercise for the reader (see Exercise 2.4).

An example of (2.4) for a non-Gaussian response is the following simple logistic regression model involving a single explanatory variable, x:

$$\text{logit}[\Pr(Y_j = 1 | U)] = \beta_0 + \beta_1 x_j + \alpha U \tag{2.8}$$

where $U \sim N(0, 1)$. Here the regression parameter β_1 again represents a change in the log odds per unit change in x, but this is now conditional on the subject's own value of U. Simulation of the simple model in (2.8) allows us to illustrate the different meanings of the regression parameters in a marginal logistic regression and a conditional logistic regression model. The solid lines in Figure 2.3 show μ_j^c as functions of x for each of 20 individuals, whilst the dotted line shows μ_j calculated as the average of the individual specific functions. It is, in effect, the dotted line that we would be estimating in a marginal model. A marginal regression model does not address questions concerning heterogeneity between subjects.

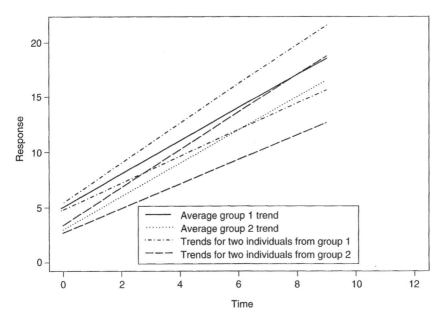

Figure 2.2 Graphical illustration of random intercept and slope model.

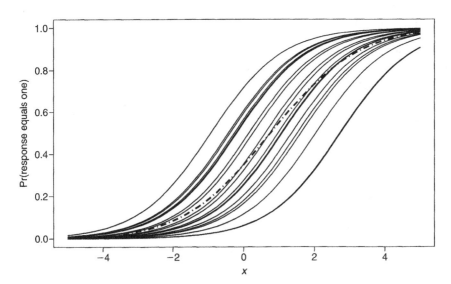

Figure 2.3 Simulation of the probability of a positive response in a random intercept logistic regression model for 20 subjects. The dotted line is the average over all 20 subjects.

Estimating the parameters in a random effects model is again generally undertaken by maximum likelihood. The likelihood contains an integral over the unobserved random effects of the joint distribution of the data and the random effects – see Everitt and Pickles (2000) for details. For normally distributed responses this presents no real problems, but for non-normal responses numerical integration techniques are necessary to evaluate the likelihood, and most commercially available software can only deal with very simple models for such variables. Software suitable for fitting more complex models is, however, available and is detailed at the end of the chapter.

Transition models

In a transition GLM, correlation amongst the observations is assumed to arise from the dependence of the present observation on one or more past values. For this type of model interest lies in the conditional mean at a fixed time, given the history of the responses to that point. Here we model the mean and variance of the response at time j conditionally on past responses $y_{j-1}, y_{j-2}, \ldots$. The essentials of our GLM in this case become:

$$g(\mu_j^t) = \beta_0 + \beta_1 x_{1j} + \beta_2 x_{2j} + \cdots + \beta_q x_{qj} + \alpha_1 y_{j-1}$$
$$+ \alpha_2 y_{j-2} + \cdots + \alpha_r y_{j-r} \qquad (2.9)$$

$$V_j^t = \phi V(\mu) \qquad (2.10)$$

where now μ_j^t and V_j^t are the expectation and variance of the response on the jth occasion, conditional on $y_{j-1}, \ldots, y_{j-r}$. The integer r is called the *order* of the model. (Fitting such a transition model is only sensible where data are collected at regularly spaced times common to all individuals in the study, a restriction not necessary for random effects models.)

Transition models can be fitted by maximizing the conditional likelihood of $y_2, \ldots, y_m$ given y_1; for details, see Diggle *et al.* (1994). No special software is necessary. Examples of the application of transition models are given in Everitt and Pickles (2000), but the need to condition on the initial response means that these models are of limited value for short series, and there are also problems associated with fitting transition models of higher order. Consequently, we shall not discuss such models further, instead concentrating on the more useful marginal and random effects models.

2.3 Marginal and conditional regression models for continuous responses with Gaussian errors

To illustrate the generalized linear models suitable for longitudinal data described in the previous section, we begin by considering the most straightforward case, namely where the response is continuous and the conditional normality assumption is likely to be justified. Assuming normality means that maximum likelihood estimation is possible. In this case the models described in Section 2.2 are essentially equivalent to one another if they assume the same correlation structure; see Diggle *et al.* (1994).

To illustrate the use of both marginal and random effects models for such response measures we shall use the data shown in Table 2.1. These data arise from a study investigating the effects of various doses of an anaesthetic on post-surgical recovery amongst children. Sixty young children undergoing surgery were randomized to receive one of four doses (15, 20, 25 and 30 mg/kg); 15 children were assigned to each dose. Recovery scores were assigned upon admission to the recovery room and at 10,

Table 2.1 Anaesthesia recovery data

Dose (mg/kg)	Subject	Age (months)	Duration of surgery (minutes)	Recovery score, by time (min) after surgery			
				0	10	20	30
15	1	36	128	3	5	6	6
15	2	35	70	3	4	6	6
15	3	54	138	1	1	1	4
15	4	47	67	1	3	3	5
15	5	42	55	5	6	6	6
15	6	35	94	3	3	6	6
15	7	30	44	6	6	6	6
15	8	57	54	1	1	1	6
15	9	30	74	1	1	4	6
15	10	41	65	2	2	2	2
15	11	34	50	1	3	3	5
15	12	62	35	3	3	5	6
15	13	24	55	1	1	1	4
15	14	39	165	1	3	5	5
15	15	66	158	0	2	2	3
20	16	22	75	1	1	1	6
20	17	49	42	1	1	1	6
20	18	36	58	2	3	3	6
20	19	43	60	1	1	2	3
20	20	23	64	5	6	6	6
20	21	30	46	1	1	2	4
20	22	9	114	6	6	6	6
20	23	14	50	4	4	6	6
20	24	2	95	1	4	5	5
20	25	50	125	1	2	2	5
20	26	26	127	6	6	6	6
20	27	40	173	0	0	0	4
20	28	12	110	3	6	6	6
20	29	42	47	1	1	5	6
20	30	18	97	2	2	3	5
25	31	26	103	1	1	0	3
25	32	28	89	3	6	6	6
25	33	41	51	2	3	4	4
25	34	46	93	1	1	5	6
25	35	37	45	2	3	6	6
25	36	28	68	6	6	6	6
25	37	37	35	3	5	6	6
25	38	60	54	2	3	3	6
25	39	60	55	1	1	1	3
25	40	38	78	0	2	6	6
25	41	47	118	0	0	0	0
25	42	38	98	1	1	1	4
25	43	23	58	1	2	6	6
25	44	56	190	1	1	1	1
25	45	31	125	0	3	5	6
30	46	46	72	4	6	6	6
30	47	38	85	2	4	6	6
30	48	59	54	4	5	5	6
30	49	16	100	1	1	1	1
30	50	65	113	2	3	3	5

(Continued)

Table 2.1   (*Continued*)

Dose (mg/kg)	Subject	Age (months)	Duration of surgery (minutes)	Recovery score, by time (min) after surgery			
				0	10	20	30
30	51	53	72	3	4	4	6
30	52	50	70	0	5	5	5
30	53	13	85	0	0	0	4
30	54	17	25	0	0	0	0
30	55	70	53	1	1	1	4
30	56	13	45	0	0	4	6
30	57	60	41	1	1	4	6
30	58	12	61	1	1	4	6
30	59	27	61	3	5	5	6
30	60	56	106	0	1	1	3

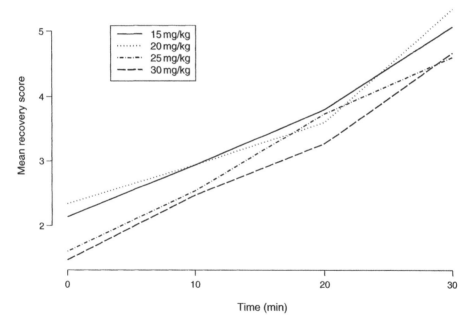

Figure 2.4   Mean profiles of recovery scores for four drug doses – data in Table 2.1.

20, and 30 minutes following admission. The response at each of the four time points was recorded on a six-point scale ranging from 0 (least favourable) to 6 (most favourable). In addition to the dosage, potential covariates were age of patient (in months) and duration of surgery (in minutes).

It is sensible to begin our examination of these data by looking at some relevant plots. A plot of mean profiles of recovery scores by dosage groups is shown in Figure 2.4, and boxplots of the observations at each time point for each treatment group are given

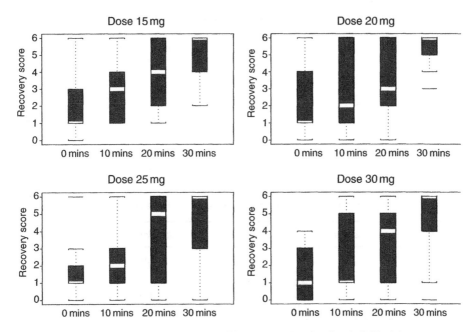

Figure 2.5   Boxplots of recovery scores for different drug doses – data in Table 2.1.

in Figure 2.5. The four dose mean profiles in Figure 2.4 all show an increase in recovery score with time. In general, recovery seems best at all times with the lowest dose of anaesthetic and worst with the largest dose, although differences are not great. The boxplots in Figure 2.5 suggest that the variance of recovery scores changes with time, and that at some time points the recovery scores are considerably skewed.

To begin our formal analysis of these data, we shall fit a GLM that includes linear effects for age, dose, duration and time. We assume an identity link function and Gaussian errors, despite the contraindications in Figure 2.5. We shall also assume, unrealistically, that the repeated measurements on each child are independent of one another. Such an analysis can be carried out using a GLM approach after organizing the data so that there is one response measure per record, with each subject contributing as many records as repeated measures. For example, the recovery data for the first two subjects rearranged in this way are shown in Table 2.2. Organized in this way the whole data set would consist of 240 records.

The results from this analysis are given in Table 2.3. The drop in deviance associated with including the four explanatory variables suggests that at least some of the covariates are predictive of recovery. The z statistics indicate that the time effect noted in Figure 2.4 is highly significant and that each of the other three covariates may also be associated with recovery. We have not investigated in this analysis whether, say, a time $\times$ dose interaction is needed in this model, but leave it as an exercise for the reader (see Exercise 2.1).

We shall not dwell further on the results in Table 2.3 since they were derived under the unconvincing assumption that the four repeated measurements are independent; as mentioned earlier, this is likely to mean that the parameter standard errors in particular will be poorly estimated. The bootstrap and sandwich estimator approaches could

Table 2.2   Anaesthesia recovery data for the first two children, after reorganization

Subject	Dose	Age	Duration	Time	Score
1	15	36	128	0	3
1	15	36	128	10	5
1	15	36	128	20	6
1	15	36	128	30	6
2	15	35	70	0	3
2	15	35	70	10	4
2	15	35	70	20	6
2	15	35	70	30	6

Table 2.3   Results from independence model with Gaussian errors for recovery data

Covariate	Estimated regression parameter	Standard error	Estimate/SE
Intercept	4.115	0.647	6.356
Time	0.099	0.010	9.539
Dose	−0.045	0.021	−2.142
Age	−0.017	0.007	−2.382
Duration	−0.008	0.003	−2.563

(Dispersion parameter for Gaussian family taken to be 3.286.)
Null deviance: 1126.30 on 239 degrees of freedom.
Residual deviance: 772.21 on 235 degrees of freedom.

be used to obtain better estimates, but we prefer to leave giving an example of these approaches until later. Here we will move on to consider models for the recovery data that specify a more realistic correlational structure for the repeated responses.

As a first step away from the naïve assumption of independence, we shall consider an exchangeable correlation structure for the four repeated recovery scores. Here the assumptions are that all the responses at each time point have the same variance, and that all pairs of repeated measures have the same correlation. The graphical evidence of Figure 2.3 suggests that the first assumption is questionable, and intuitively it seems likely that measurements made closer together in time will be more highly correlated than those taken further apart. Nevertheless the exchangeable assumption is still likely to be an improvement on independence. The results from fitting such a model are shown in Table 2.4. The estimated regression coefficients are identical to those given in Table 2.3, but the associated standard errors for dose, age and duration are now considerably larger; the conclusion now is that there is little evidence that any of these three covariates has any effect on recovery. The estimated correlation between each pair of the repeated measures of recovery is 0.63.

Consideration of other possible correlation structures for the data is left as an exercise for readers (see Exercise 2.2), as is a more detailed investigation of which covariates should be included in a final model for the data.

The first conditional regression model to be fitted to these data is one where a simple random intercept term is included for each individual. Specifically, the model for the recovery score of the ith individual at the jth time of measurement is assumed to be

$$y_{ij} = \beta_0 + u_i + \beta_1 \text{time}_j + \beta_2 \text{age}_i + \beta_3 \text{duration}_i + \beta_4 \text{dose}_i + \varepsilon_{ij} \quad (2.11)$$

Table 2.4 Results from recovery data for Gaussian errors and exchangeable correlation structure

Covariate	Estimate regression parameter	Standard error	Estimate/SE
Intercept	4.115	1.072	3.84
Time	0.100	0.006	15.68
Dose	−0.045	0.036	−1.26
Age	−0.017	0.012	−1.40
Duration	−0.008	0.006	−1.51

Residual standard error: 1.794.
Correlation structure: compound symmetry.
Parameter estimate: rho = 0.630.

Table 2.5 Random intercept model for recovery data

Covariate	Estimated regression parameter	Standard error	Estimate/SE
Intercept	4.115	1.072	3.839
Time	0.100	0.006	15.683
Dose	−0.045	0.036	−1.260
Age	−0.017	0.012	−1.401
Duration	−0.008	0.006	−1.508

$\hat{\sigma}_u = 1.424$, $\hat{\sigma} = 1.091$; log-likelihood = −423.12.

where u_i is assumed to be normally distributed with mean zero and variance σ_u^2, and the ε_{ij} are also assumed normally distributed with mean zero and variance σ^2. Such a model implies that recovery scores at each time point have variance $\sigma_u^2 + \sigma^2$, and that the correlation between each pair of recovery scores is given by $\sigma_u^2/(\sigma_u^2 + \sigma^2)$, the compound symmetry structure as described previously. The results of fitting this random effects model are shown in Table 2.5. The estimated regression coefficients are identical to those in Tables 2.3 and 2.4, and the estimated standard errors are the same as in Table 2.4. The fitted random effects model is equivalent to the exchangeable correlation model considered earlier, and the estimated correlation for pairs of repeated measures of recovery is given by $1.42^2/(1.42^2 + 1.09^2) = 0.63$, as before.

Normal probability plots of the residuals from fitting the random intercept model, by dose group, are given in Figure 2.6. The plot shows no disturbing departure from linearity. The random effects themselves can be 'estimated' by a procedure described in Pinheiro and Bates (2000). After estimation a normal probability plot can again be used to assess their normality – see Figure 2.7. There is no evidence of any departure from the normality assumption.

More complex random effects models might be considered for these data, for example, one with both a random intercept and random slope over time for each individual:

$$y_{ij} = \beta_0 + u_{i1} + (\beta_1 + u_{i2})\text{time}_j + \beta_2\text{age}_i + \beta_3\text{duration}_i$$
$$+ \beta_4\text{dose}_i + \varepsilon_{ij} \tag{2.12}$$

where now u_{i1} and u_{i2} are assumed to have a bivariate normal distribution with mean vector the null vector, and covariance matrix

$$\Sigma = \begin{pmatrix} \sigma^2_{u_1} & \sigma_{u_1 u_2} \\ \sigma_{u_1 u_2} & \sigma^2_{u_2} \end{pmatrix}$$

The results from fitting the model specified in (2.12) are given in Table 2.6. The results are very similar to those in Table 2.5. The estimate of $\sigma^2_{u_1}$ is $1.635^2 = 2.673$, and of $\sigma^2_{u_2}$ is $0.0418^2 = 0.0017$. The estimated correlation of the two random effects is -0.472. (This apparently negative correlation between an individual's intercept and slope is largely an artefact; see Exercise 2.8.) A likelihood ratio test of whether the more complex model specified in (2.12) provides an improved fit over the random intercept model takes the value 10.03, with an associated p-value of 0.007. The random intercept and slope model does describe the data better than the simpler random intercept model, although the conclusions about the effects of the covariates remain largely the same for both models.

2.4   Marginal and conditional regression models for non-normal responses

In this section we consider the types of regression models for longitudinal data introduced in Section 2.2, for the more interesting case of non-normal responses, in particular binary and count type responses. We begin with a data set involving the former; the data shown in Table 2.7 were collected in a clinical trial comparing two treatments for a respiratory illness (Davis, 1991). In each of two centres, eligible patients were randomly assigned to active treatment or placebo. Each participant's respiratory status (categorized as 0 = poor, 1 = good) was determined at each of four monthly visits.

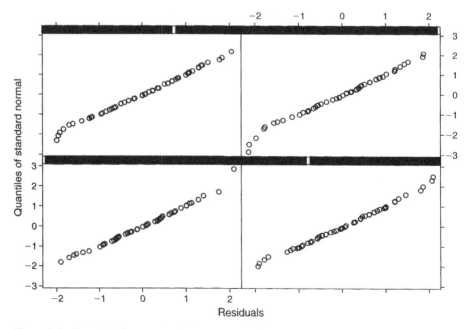

Figure 2.6   Residuals from random intercept model fitted to surgical recovery data.

To begin, we shall fit a logistic regression model to these data using standard GLM software by simply assuming independence for the repeated measurements of respiratory status. Again the data need to be arranged with one response measure per record with each subject contributing as many records as repeated measures. The model to be considered is

$$\text{logit}[p_j] = \beta_0 + \beta_1 \text{treatment} + \beta_2 \text{time}_j + \beta_3 \text{sex} + \beta_4 \text{age}$$
$$+ \beta_5 \text{centre} + \beta_6 \text{baseline} \qquad (2.13)$$

where p_j is the expected or average value of the response on the jth occasion, and treatment, sex, and centre represent dummy variables coding these factors. The results of fitting the model are summarized in Table 2.8. Treatment, baseline, centre and to a lesser extent, age, appear to affect a child's respiratory status. The estimated regression coefficients are interpreted as log odds ratios in the usual way. Exponentiating the

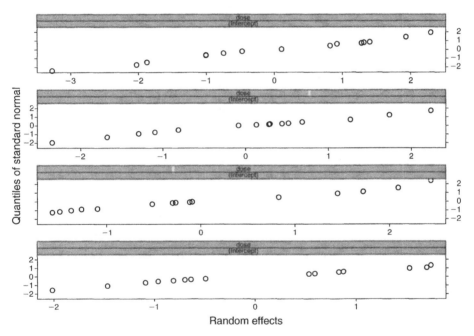

Figure 2.7 Normal probability plot of estimated random effects in model fitted to surgical recovery data.

Table 2.6 Random intercept and slope model for recovery data

Covariate	Estimated regression parameter	Standard error	Estimate/SE
Intercept	4.125	1.073	3.843
Time	0.100	0.008	12.852
Dose	−0.045	0.036	−1.247
Age	−0.017	0.012	−1.385
Duration	−0.009	0.006	−1.582

$\hat{\sigma}_{u_1} = 1.636$, $\hat{\sigma}_{u_2} = 0.042$, $\hat{\rho}_{u_1 u_2} = -0.472$, $\hat{\sigma} = 0.948$; log-likelihood $= -418.11$.

Table 2.7　Respiratory disorder data (Taken with permission of Wiley from Davies, 1991.)

Patient	Centre	Treatment	Sex	Age	BL	V1	V2	V3	V4
1	1	1	1	46	0	0	0	0	0
2	1	1	1	28	0	0	0	0	0
3	1	2	1	23	1	1	1	1	1
4	1	1	1	44	1	1	1	1	0
5	1	1	2	13	1	1	1	1	1
6	1	2	1	34	0	0	0	0	0
7	1	1	1	43	0	1	0	1	1
8	1	2	1	28	0	0	0	0	0
9	1	2	1	31	1	1	1	1	1
10	1	1	1	37	1	0	1	1	0
11	1	2	1	30	1	1	1	1	1
12	1	2	1	14	0	1	1	1	0
13	1	1	1	23	1	1	0	0	0
14	1	1	1	30	0	0	0	0	0
15	1	1	1	20	1	1	1	1	1
16	1	2	1	22	0	0	0	0	1
17	1	1	1	25	0	0	0	0	0
18	1	2	2	47	0	0	1	1	1
19	1	1	2	31	0	0	0	0	0
20	1	2	1	20	1	1	0	1	0
21	1	2	1	26	0	1	0	1	0
22	1	2	1	46	1	1	1	1	1
23	1	2	1	32	1	1	1	1	1
24	1	2	1	48	0	1	0	0	0
25	1	1	2	35	0	0	0	0	0
26	1	2	1	26	0	0	0	0	0
27	1	1	1	23	1	1	0	1	1
28	1	1	2	36	0	1	1	0	0
29	1	1	1	19	0	1	1	0	0
30	1	2	1	28	0	0	0	0	0
31	1	1	1	37	0	0	0	0	0
32	1	2	1	23	0	1	1	1	1
33	1	2	1	30	1	1	1	1	0
34	1	1	1	15	0	0	1	1	0
35	1	2	1	26	0	0	0	1	0
36	1	1	2	45	0	0	0	0	0
37	1	2	1	31	0	0	1	0	0
38	1	2	1	50	0	0	0	0	0
39	1	1	1	28	0	0	0	0	0
40	1	1	1	26	0	0	0	0	0
41	1	1	1	14	0	0	0	0	1
42	1	2	1	31	0	0	1	0	0
43	1	1	1	13	1	1	1	1	1
44	1	1	1	27	0	0	0	0	0
45	1	1	1	26	0	1	0	1	1
46	1	1	1	49	0	0	0	0	0
47	1	1	1	63	0	0	0	0	0
48	1	2	1	57	1	1	1	1	1
49	1	1	1	27	1	1	1	1	1
50	1	2	1	22	0	0	1	1	1
51	1	2	1	15	0	0	1	1	1
52	1	1	1	43	0	0	0	1	0
53	1	2	2	32	0	0	0	1	0

(Continued)

Table 2.7 (*Continued*)

Patient	Centre	Treatment	Sex	Age	BL	V1	V2	V3	V4
54	1	2	1	11	1	1	1	1	0
55	1	1	1	24	1	1	1	1	1
56	1	2	1	25	0	1	1	0	1
57	2	1	2	39	0	0	0	0	0
58	2	2	1	25	0	0	1	1	1
59	2	2	1	58	1	1	1	1	1
60	2	1	2	51	1	1	0	1	1
61	2	1	2	32	1	0	0	1	1
62	2	1	1	45	1	1	0	0	0
63	2	1	2	44	1	1	1	1	1
64	2	1	2	48	0	0	0	0	0
65	2	2	1	26	0	1	1	1	1
66	2	2	1	14	0	1	1	1	1
67	2	1	2	48	0	0	0	0	0
68	2	2	1	13	1	1	1	1	1
69	2	1	1	20	0	1	1	1	1
70	2	2	1	37	1	1	0	0	1
71	2	2	1	25	1	1	1	1	1
72	2	2	1	20	0	0	0	0	0
73	2	1	2	58	0	1	0	0	0
74	2	1	1	38	1	1	0	0	0
75	2	2	1	55	1	1	1	1	1
76	2	2	1	24	1	1	1	1	1
77	2	1	2	36	1	1	0	0	1
78	2	1	1	36	0	1	1	1	1
79	2	2	2	60	1	1	1	1	1
80	2	1	1	15	1	0	0	1	1
81	2	2	1	25	1	1	1	1	0
82	2	2	1	35	1	1	1	1	1
83	2	2	1	19	1	1	0	1	1
84	2	1	2	31	1	1	1	1	1
85	2	2	1	21	1	1	1	1	1
86	2	2	2	37	0	1	1	1	1
87	2	1	1	52	0	1	1	1	1
88	2	2	1	55	0	0	1	1	0
89	2	1	1	19	1	0	0	1	1
90	2	1	1	20	1	0	1	1	1
91	2	1	1	42	1	0	0	0	0
92	2	2	1	41	1	1	1	1	1
93	2	2	1	52	0	0	0	0	0
94	2	1	2	47	0	1	1	0	1
95	2	1	1	11	1	1	1	1	1
96	2	1	1	14	0	0	0	1	0
97	2	1	1	15	1	1	1	1	1
98	2	1	1	66	1	1	1	1	1
99	2	2	1	34	0	1	1	0	1
100	2	1	1	43	0	0	0	0	0
101	2	1	1	33	1	1	1	0	1
102	2	1	1	48	1	1	0	0	0
103	2	2	1	20	0	1	1	1	1
104	2	1	2	39	1	0	1	0	0
105	2	2	1	28	0	1	0	0	0
106	2	1	2	38	0	0	0	0	0

(*Continued*)

Table 2.7   (*Continued*)

Patient	Centre	Treatment	Sex	Age	BL	V1	V2	V3	V4
107	2	2	1	43	1	1	1	1	1
108	2	2	2	39	0	1	1	1	1
109	2	2	1	68	0	1	1	1	1
110	2	2	2	63	1	1	1	1	1
111	2	2	1	31	1	1	1	1	1

Treatment: 1 = placebo, 2 = active.
Sex: 1 = male, 2 = female.
Source: Davis (1991).

Table 2.8   Logistic regression model for respiratory disorder data assuming responses are independent

Covariate	Estimated regression parameter	Standard error	Robust SE	Bootstrap SE
Treatment	1.301	0.237	0.349	0.392
Time	−0.064	0.100	0.082	0.080
Sex	0.119	0.295	0.443	0.453
Age	−1.819	0.887	1.305	1.459
Baseline	1.884	0.241	0.349	0.366
Centre	0.672	0.240	0.355	0.355

(Dispersion parameter for binomial family taken to be 1.)
Null deviance: 608.93 on 443 degrees of freedom.
Residual deviance: 482.80 on 437 degrees of freedom.

regression coefficients will give the effects in terms of odds ratios themselves. For treatment group, for example, this leads to a 95% confidence interval for the odds ratio of (2.307, 5.842); active treatment clearly results in an improved chance of a child having a good respiratory status.

The independence assumption for these data is, of course, simplistic. Here we shall try to get some idea of how misleading it might be by comparing the standard errors of the parameters given in Table 2.8 with those calculated by the sandwich estimator, and by the use of the bootstrap approach. The resulting standard errors are also shown in Table 2.8 alongside the corresponding estimates from the independence assumption. The bootstrap and robust standard errors are relatively close to one another, and, for all but the time effect, considerably larger than the independence standard errors. For the time effect the reverse is the case. Using the robust standard error for treatment group now leads to a 95% confidence interval for the conditional odds ratio of (1.852, 7.276), considerably wider than the interval given above.

Next we consider the use of the GEE approach to fit marginal models to the respiratory data under a variety of assumptions about their correlational structure. Results are given in Table 2.9 for a model with only treatment and time as covariates. Robust standard errors are also given. Here the differences between the two standard error estimates are smaller than in Table 2.8, as is to be expected since, unlike the independence working model used there, these models all make at least a plausible assumption as to the correlation structure. (Marked differences in the model standard error estimates and the robust values would again have suggested possible model misspecification.)

Table 2.9   Results from fitting a logistic regression model to the respiratory status data under various assumptions about correlational structure

Covariate	Model	Estimate	Classical		Robust	
			SE	Estimate/SE	SE	Estimate/SE
Treatment	Exch	1.256	0.331	3.79	0.348	3.61
	AR-1	1.205	0.308	3.91	0.349	3.45
	Unstr	1.239	0.330	3.76	0.347	3.58
Time	Exch	−0.078	0.081	−0.97	0.082	−0.95
	AR-1	−0.097	0.101	−0.96	0.083	−1.18
	Unstr	−0.086	0.085	−1.01	0.082	−1.05

Table 2.10   Estimated correlation matrices for the respiratory status data

(a) Exchangeable

$$\hat{\mathbf{R}} = \begin{pmatrix} 1.00 & & & \\ 0.33 & 1.00 & & \\ 0.33 & 0.33 & 1.00 & \\ 0.33 & 0.33 & & 1.00 \end{pmatrix}$$

(b) AR-1

$$\hat{\mathbf{R}} = \begin{pmatrix} 1.00 & & & \\ 0.38 & 1.00 & & \\ 0.15 & 0.38 & 1.00 & \\ 0.06 & 0.15 & 0.38 & 1.00 \end{pmatrix}$$

(c) Unstructured

$$\hat{\mathbf{R}} = \begin{pmatrix} 1.00 & & & \\ 0.32 & 1.00 & & \\ 0.20 & 0.42 & 1.00 & \\ 0.29 & 0.34 & 0.38 & 1.00 \end{pmatrix}$$

Table 2.10 gives the lower triangle of the estimated correlation matrices from each of these models. The estimated correlations from the unstructured model appear to be closer to those of an exchangeable structure than the autoregressive (AR-1) structure. In the latter model, the correlation between pairs of observations is expected to decline with separation in time much more quickly than it actually appears to do, whereas the exchangeable model assumes that this correlation remains constant. This greater similarity, in this case, of the unstructured and exchangeable models, as compared to the AR-1 model, is also reflected in the estimated regression coefficients and standard errors.

We now consider some random effects models for the respiratory data, beginning with the following simple model for p_{ij}, the expected value of the response for the ith

Table 2.11   Results from the random intercept logistic regression model fitted to the respiratory status data

Covariate	Estimated regression parameter	Standard error	Estimate/SE
Treatment	2.13	0.563	3.79
Visit	−0.10	0.126	−0.81
Sex	0.20	0.686	0.29
Age	−0.025	0.021	−1.20
Baseline	3.04	0.606	5.02
Centre	1.04	0.562	1.86

Estimated variance of random effects = 4.12, with standard error 0.33.

individual on the jth occasion, given the value of the random effect associated with the individual:

$$\text{logit}(p_{ij}|U) = \beta_0 + \beta_1 \text{treatment}_i + \beta_2 \text{time}_j + \beta_3 \text{sex}_i + \beta_4 \text{age}_i$$
$$+ \beta_5 \text{centre}_i + \beta_6 \text{baseline}_i + U_i \qquad (2.14)$$

The results from fitting this model are shown in Table 2.11. The significance of the effects as estimated in (2.11) and by a corresponding GEE model is generally similar. However, as expected from previous discussion, and unlike the Gaussian error situation of the previous section, the estimated coefficients are substantially larger. Thus, while the estimated effect of treatment given the set of observed covariates in (2.14) was estimated by a marginal model with an exchangeable correlation structure to increase the log odds of being disease free by 1.3, the estimate from the random effects model is 2.13. These are not inconsistent results but reflect the fact that the models are estimating different parameters. The random effects estimator is conditional upon each patient's random effect, a quantity that is rarely known in practice. It represents the effect of treatment on a given participant, whereas the marginal effect is the average effect in the population. Were we to examine the log odds of the average predicted probabilities with and without treatment (averaged over the random effect), this would give an estimate comparable to that estimated within the marginal model.

In terms of covariate effects, the parameterization of this random effects model corresponds to the marginal model considered earlier in this section (the model in (2.13)). The model is, however, now a model of the *joint* responses. The difference is highlighted by tabulating the observed frequencies of each pattern of responses along with the values predicted by each model – see Table 2.12. Typical of such data, the sequences with a preponderance of one type of response are more common than expected under the assumption of independence, and the sequences with alternating responses considerably fewer. The introduction of the random effect has captured the pattern of persistence in response remarkably well.

The results of fitting a further random effects model to the respiratory data, one with both a random intercept and random slope, are shown in Table 2.13. The conclusions remain the same as those arrived at from the random intercept model.

Finally in this chapter, we shall consider some models for the data set shown in Table 2.14. These data were originally given by Thall and Vail (1990) and arise from a clinical trial of treatment for epilepsy in which a total of 59 patients were randomly allocated to either a placebo or the active treatment, here the drug progabide. In this trial, the response variable was a count of the number of seizures within four successive

Table 2.12 Sample frequencies and predicted frequencies for respiratory status data

Response	Observed frequency	Independence working model	Random effects model
Baseline 0			
0000	25	13.3	21.9
0001	2	4.3	3.1
0010	4	4.6	3.5
0011	0	2.3	1.4
0100	2	5.0	4.0
0101	0	2.5	1.6
0110	2	2.7	1.8
0111	4	2.1	1.7
1000	3	5.4	4.5
1001	0	2.7	1.8
1010	1	2.9	2.0
1011	2	2.2	1.9
1100	2	3.2	2.2
1101	3	2.4	1.6
1110	1	2.6	2.1
1111	10	2.7	3.2
Baseline 1			
0000	1	0.3	0.2
0001	0	0.5	0.3
0010	0	0.6	0.3
0011	3	1.2	0.6
0100	1	0.6	0.6
0101	0	1.3	0.9
0110	1	1.4	0.9
0111	1	4.0	2.4
1000	4	0.7	1.1
1001	2	1.4	1.8
1010	1	1.5	1.6
1011	3	4.3	3.9
1100	0	1.6	3.1
1101	1	4.6	5.7
1110	5	5.0	5.5
1111	27	21.0	21.2

Table 2.13 Results from the random intercepts and slope logistic regression model fitted to the respiratory status data

Covariate	Estimated regression parameter	Standard error	Estimate/SE
Treat	2.135	0.564	3.78
Time	−0.102	0.126	−0.81
Sex	0.198	0.691	0.29
Age	−0.025	0.021	−1.21
Baseline	3.037	0.602	5.04
Centre	1.043	0.561	1.86

intervals of two weeks. A baseline measure of the response was also taken and, in addition, the age of each patient was recorded.

We begin by fitting a Poisson regression model under the assumption that the repeated counts available on each patient are independent. Again this involves nothing

Table 2.14   Data from a clinical trial of patients suffering from epilepsy (Taken with permission of the Biometrics Society from Thall and Vail, 1990.)

Subject ID	Period 1	Period 2	Period 3	Period 4	Treatment	Baseline	Age
1	5	3	3	3	0	11	31
2	3	5	3	3	0	11	30
3	2	4	0	5	0	6	25
4	4	4	1	4	0	8	36
5	7	18	9	21	0	66	22
6	5	2	8	7	0	27	29
7	6	4	0	2	0	12	31
8	40	20	23	12	0	52	42
9	5	6	6	5	0	23	37
10	14	13	6	0	0	10	28
11	26	12	6	22	0	52	36
12	12	6	8	4	0	33	24
13	4	4	6	2	0	18	23
14	7	9	12	14	0	42	36
15	16	24	10	9	0	87	26
16	11	0	0	5	0	50	26
17	0	0	3	3	0	18	28
18	37	29	28	29	0	111	31
19	3	5	2	5	0	18	32
20	3	0	6	7	0	20	21
21	3	4	3	4	0	12	29
22	3	4	3	4	0	9	21
23	2	3	3	5	0	17	32
24	8	12	2	8	0	28	25
25	18	24	76	25	0	55	30
26	2	1	2	1	0	9	40
27	3	1	4	2	0	10	19
28	13	15	13	12	0	47	22
29	11	14	9	8	1	76	18
30	8	7	9	4	1	38	32
31	0	4	3	0	1	19	20
32	3	6	1	3	1	10	30
33	2	6	7	4	1	19	18
34	4	3	1	3	1	24	24
35	22	17	19	16	1	31	30
36	5	4	7	4	1	14	35
37	2	4	0	4	1	11	27
38	3	7	7	7	1	67	20
39	4	18	2	5	1	41	22
40	2	1	1	0	1	7	28
41	0	2	4	0	1	22	23
42	5	4	0	3	1	13	40
43	11	14	25	15	1	46	33
44	10	5	3	8	1	36	21
45	19	7	6	7	1	38	35
46	1	1	2	3	1	7	25
47	6	10	8	8	1	36	26
48	2	1	0	0	1	11	25
49	102	65	72	63	1	151	22
50	4	3	2	4	1	22	32
51	8	6	5	7	1	41	25
52	1	3	1	5	1	32	35

(*Continued*)

Table 2.14   (*Continued*)

Subject ID	Period 1	Period 2	Period 3	Period 4	Treatment	Baseline	Age
53	18	11	28	13	1	56	21
54	6	3	4	0	1	24	41
55	3	5	4	3	1	16	32
56	1	23	19	8	1	22	26
57	2	3	0	1	1	25	21
58	0	0	0	0	1	13	36
59	1	4	3	2	1	12	37

Table 2.15   Poisson regression model fitted to the epilepsy data assuming independence

Covariate	Estimated regression parameter	Standard error	Estimate/SE
Intercept	0.707	0.144	4.904
Time	−0.029	0.010	−2.896
Age	0.023	0.004	5.654
Treat	−0.153	0.048	−3.196
BL	0.023	0.006	44.486

(Dispersion parameter for Poisson family taken to be 1.)
Null deviance: 2522.8 on 235 degrees of freedom.
Residual deviance: 950.1 on 231 degrees of freedom.

Table 2.16   Poisson regression models fitted to the epilepsy data: results for three correlational structures

Coefficient	Estimated regression parameter	Standard error	Estimate/SE
Exchangeable			
Treat	−0.148	0.071	−2.08
BL	0.023	0.008	30.10
Age	0.024	0.006	3.95
Time	−0.059	0.016	−3.74
AR−1			
Treat	−0.164	0.068	−2.40
BL	0.023	0.001	32.02
Age	0.026	0.006	4.54
Time	−0.064	0.020	−3.20
Unstructured			
Treat	−0.149	0.067	−2.22
BL	0.023	0.001	31.84
Age	0.024	0.006	4.16
Time	−0.051	0.018	−2.85

more difficult than a rearrangement of the data and the use of standard GLM software. The results of fitting this model are shown in Table 2.15. The unrealistic assumption of independence makes the results in Table 2.15 less than convincing. Consequently, Table 2.16 gives the results obtained from fitting a series of models with more realistic assumptions about the correlational structure of the repeated measurements.

The treatment effect, whilst remaining significant, is less so than in the independence model. The same is true for other covariates. There remains the problem of likely overdispersion in these data which needs to be dealt with. This is left as an exercise for readers (see Exercise 2.6).

2.5   Summary

Longitudinal data occur frequently in medical research and can now be appropriately analysed using a variety of methods. For assumed Gaussian responses, the estimated parameters from all types of models can be made to have a similar interpretation. But this is not so for non-normal responses, where the different modelling approaches do not attempt to estimate the same effect. Marginal models are straightforward to apply and do estimate effects that are seemingly of immediate interest in most applications. Currently there is a strong preference for the use of marginal models since population average effects are generally most useful in assessing the implications of results for public health. But some authors, for example, Lindsey and Lambert (1998), have questioned the value of the parameter estimates from such models. Certainly the case for marginal models is not so overwhelming that they should be used to the exclusion of others.

The methods described in this chapter can also be used in other situations where responses are likely to be correlated, for example, when individuals are samples from families or geographical regions. A distinguishing feature of such 'clustered' data is that they are likely to exhibit intraclass correlation, analogous to that arising from the repeated measures collected in a longitudinal study as described in this chapter.

Software

Again a wide variety of software is available for fitting the types of models described in this chapter. But in this case it may be necessary to search a little wider than the standard packages to find suitable programs for *all* the analyses described. Examples of relevant procedures are as follows:

SAS   `proc mixed` (for random effects models);
         `proc genmod` (for generalized estimating equations).
STATA   `xtgee` command (for generalized estimating equations);
         `xtreg` command (for random effects models with a Gaussian response);
         `xtlogit` command (for a simple random intercept logistic regression).
         To fit more complex random effects models to non-normal longitudinal data the STATA program `gllamm`, developed by Dr Sophia Rabe-Hesketh, can be used. The program and manual can be downloaded from http://www.iop.kcl.ac.uk/iop/departments/biocomp/programs/gllamm. html
S-PLUS   `gls` function (for longitudinal data with a Gaussian response);
         `lme` function (for random effects models with a Gaussian response).

MLWIN

A generalized estimating equation function is not included in S-PLUS 2000 or S-PLUS 6, but one is available from
http://www.stats.ox.ac.uk/pub/SWin
Very useful package for fitting random effects models to longitudinal data involving either continuous or binary response variables: see
http://multilevel.ioe.ac.uk/index.html

Full details of how to use the first three of these packages in the analysis of longitudinal data are given in Der and Everitt (2001), Rabe-Hesketh and Everitt (2000) and Everitt (2001b). Software for fitting generalized estimating regression models is reviewed in Horton and Lipsitz (1999). Software for fitting random effects models is reviewed in Zhou *et al.* (1999).

Exercises

2.1 Investigate whether a time × dose interaction is needed when modelling the recovery data in Table 2.1. Also explore the need for a quadratic effect of time.

2.2 Find bootstrap and sandwich estimates of the standard errors of the parameters in the independence model for the recovery data fitted in Section 2.3. What do they suggest about the independence model?

2.3 Fit models to the recovery data with other than independent or exchangeable correlation structures. How do the results compare with those given in the text?

2.4 What type of structure for the covariance matrix between the repeated responses does the random intercept and slope model specified in equation (2.7) imply?

2.5 In the random intercept and slope model fitted to the recovery data in Section 2.3, the estimated covariance between the random intercept and slope terms was -0.472. Fit a model which sets the covariance to zero and test whether there is any evidence of a non-zero covariance.

2.6 Compare the results given in the text for the treatment of epilepsy data with those from treating the response as Gaussian.

2.7 Investigate the possible overdispersion problem in the epilepsy data.

2.8 Refit the random intercept and slope model to the recovery data using time minus its mean value as covariate rather than simply time, and examine what happens to the estimated correlation between the intercept and slope random effects. Explain.

3

Missing Values, Drop-outs, Compliance and Intention-to-Treat

3.1 Introduction

In the previous chapter several methods suitable for the modelling of longitudinal data were described. In the context of medicine, most longitudinal data arise from clinical trials, and the examples used in Chapter 2 reflect this. But these examples, useful though they were for illustrating various aspects of the modelling process, were unrealistic in the sense that none of them suffered from any of the problems that generally confront analysers of trial data, for example, missing values, drop-outs and non-compliance. Consequently, these matters are taken up in this chapter.

3.2 Missing values and drop-outs

In a clinical trial comparing two treatments for maternal pain relief during labour, 83 women in labour were randomized to receive an experimental pain medication (43 subjects) or placebo (40 subjects). Treatment was initiated when the cervical dilation was 8 cm. At 30 min intervals, the amount of pain was self-reported by placing a mark on a 100 mm line (0 = no pain, 100 = very much pain). The resulting data are shown in Table 3.1.

A notable difference between the data from this study and the data sets analysed in Chapter 2 is that the six intended measures of pain are not made on all the women in the trial; the data set contains many *missing values*. In longitudinal studies, missing values may occur intermittently, or they may arise because a participant 'drops out' of the study before the end as specified in the protocol. Dropping out of a study implies that once an observation at a particular time point is missing so are all the remaining planned observations. Many studies will contain missing values of both types, although Table 3.1 only contains the latter, and in practice it is missing values that result from participants dropping out that cause most problems when coming to analyse the resulting data set. The very best way to avoid problems with missing values is not to have any! But in this less than ideal world this is frequently not possible and we are then faced with the problem

Table 3.1   Self-reported pain scores at 30 min intervals for 83 women in labour

Patient	30	60	90	120	150	180
1	0.0	0.0	0.0	NA	NA	NA
2	0.0	0.0	0.0	2.5	2.3	14.0
3	5.0	1.0	1.0	0.0	5.0	NA
4	48.0	85.0	0.0	0.0	NA	NA
5	5.0	NA	NA	NA	NA	NA
6	0.0	0.0	0.0	NA	NA	NA
7	42.0	42.0	45.0	NA	NA	NA
8	0.0	0.0	0.0	0.0	6.0	24.0
9	35.0	13.0	NA	NA	NA	NA
10	30.5	81.5	67.5	98.5	97.0	NA
11	44.5	55.0	69.0	72.5	39.5	26.0
12	0.0	0.0	0.0	0.0	0.0	0.0
13	30.5	26.0	24.0	29.0	45.0	91.0
14	6.5	7.0	4.0	10.0	NA	NA
15	8.5	19.5	16.5	42.5	45.5	48.5
16	9.5	7.5	5.5	4.5	0.0	7.0
17	10.0	18.0	32.5	0.0	0.0	0.0
18	20.5	32.5	37.0	39.0	NA	NA
19	91.5	4.5	32.0	10.5	10.5	10.5
20	0.0	0.0	0.0	13.5	7.0	NA
21	0.0	0.0	1.0	1.5	0.0	0.0
22	21.0	15.5	10.5	11.5	11.0	9.5
23	4.0	19.5	22.0	57.5	38.0	68.0
24	43.0	43.0	41.5	41.5	NA	NA
25	0.0	0.0	0.0	0.0	0.0	1.5
26	0.0	0.0	0.0	0.0	0.0	0.0
27	0.0	35.0	72.0	NA	NA	NA
28	19.0	23.0	0.0	37.0	42.0	66.0
29	0.0	23.0	11.0	3.0	34.5	NA
30	0.0	15.5	6.0	0.0	NA	NA
31	100.0	NA	NA	NA	NA	NA
32	3.0	NA	NA	NA	NA	NA
33	7.0	18.5	NA	NA	NA	NA
34	0.5	0.0	1.0	NA	NA	NA
35	1.0	0.0	10.0	6.0	11.0	25.0
36	9.5	14.5	9.5	2.5	23.5	63.5
37	4.5	NA	NA	NA	NA	NA
38	31.0	37.5	NA	NA	NA	NA
39	51.0	49.0	29.0	26.5	68.0	84.0
40	0.0	0.0	NA	NA	NA	NA
41	0.0	1.5	5.5	19.5	25.5	NA
42	21.0	9.0	9.0	NA	NA	NA
43	0.0	3.0	0.5	0.0	0.0	0.0
44	9.0	30.0	75.0	49.0	97.0	NA
45	0.0	1.0	27.5	95.0	100.0	NA
46	6.0	25.0	NA	NA	NA	NA
47	18.0	12.5	NA	NA	NA	NA
48	99.0	100.0	100.0	100.0	100.0	100.0
49	70.0	81.5	94.5	97.0	NA	NA
50	0.0	0.0	1.5	0.0	18.0	71.0
51	51.5	56.0	NA	NA	NA	NA
52	7.0	7.0	9.0	25.0	36.0	20.0
53	31.0	41.0	58.0	NA	NA	NA

(Continued)

Table 3.1 (*Continued*)

Patient	30	60	90	120	150	180
54	23.0	45.0	67.0	90.5	NA	NA
55	64.0	6.0	NA	NA	NA	NA
56	53.0	88.0	100.0	100.0	NA	NA
57	100.0	100.0	100.0	100.0	NA	NA
58	36.5	74.0	97.0	95.0	100.0	100.0
59	0.0	6.0	6.0	NA	NA	NA
60	79.0	80.5	85.0	90.0	97.5	97.0
61	27.5	21.0	60.0	80.0	97.0	NA
62	5.5	18.5	20.0	36.5	63.5	81.5
63	9.0	35.5	39.0	70.0	92.0	98.0
64	11.0	13.5	31.0	32.5	36.5	87.5
65	74.0	91.5	NA	NA	NA	NA
66	0.0	0.0	0.5	48.0	NA	NA
67	3.5	NA	NA	NA	NA	NA
68	2.5	5.0	33.0	52.5	89.0	96.5
69	4.5	NA	NA	NA	NA	NA
70	0.0	10.0	5.0	18.0	NA	NA
71	0.0	0.0	13.5	49.5	94.0	80.5
72	19.0	42.0	18.0	25.0	24.0	36.0
73	68.5	92.5	100.0	100.0	100.0	100.0
74	0.0	0.0	28.0	81.5	NA	100.0
75	25.0	45.5	50.0	60.5	65.5	72.5
76	100.0	NA	NA	NA	NA	NA
77	5.0	5.5	5.0	NA	NA	NA
78	26.0	35.0	42.0	94.0	97.0	97.0
79	0.0	0.0	0.0	0.0	0.0	32.0
80	0.0	NA	NA	NA	NA	NA
81	0.0	9.0	54.0	81.5	84.5	NA
82	71.0	93.0	94.0	95.0	95.0	NA
83	0.0	61.0	NA	NA	NA	NA

Patients 1–43 were in the active treatment group, 44–83 in the placebo group.
NA denotes a missing value.

of how to deal with data sets in which some of the intended observations are missing. There are four main possibilities:

- Discard incomplete cases and analyse the remainder – *complete-case analysis*.
- *Impute* or fill in the missing values and then analyse the filled-in data.
- Analyse the incomplete data by a method that does not require a complete (rectangular) data set, that is, analyse all the observed data.
- Build a model for the data that includes a component for the drop-out process.

Each of these possibilities will be discussed later, but before that we need to consider a classification of missing values first introduced by Rubin (1976), since it has implications for which approaches are suitable and which are not.

3.2.1 A classification of missing values

The pattern of missing values in a data set can be conveniently represented by a matrix, **M**, the entries of which are either zero or one, with the former indicating that

Table 3.2 Part of missing data matrix for
pain data in Table 3.1

Subject	Missing-value indicator
1	1 1 1 0 0 0
2	1 1 1 1 1 1
3	1 1 1 1 1 0
4	1 1 1 1 0 0
5	1 0 0 0 0 0
6	1 1 1 0 0 0
7	1 1 1 0 0 0
8	1 1 1 1 1 1
9	1 1 0 0 0 0
10	1 1 1 1 1 0

an intended observation is missing, and the latter that it has been made. Such a matrix has n rows and T columns, where n is the number of participants in the study and T is the number of intended measurements of the response variable. Part of the pattern matrix for the pain data in Table 3.1 is shown in Table 3.2.

We now need to consider the *missing-data mechanism*, that is, the reasons why values are missing. In particular, we need to decide whether dropping out is related to values of the response. For example, a participant in a clinical trial may be more likely to avoid a treatment and drop out of a study because she felt the treatment was ineffective, and this might be related to a poor value of the outcome measure.

In the statistical literature three types of missing values (associated in particular with dropping out) have been distinguished:

- missing completely at random (MCAR);
- missing at random (MAR);
- non-ignorable (sometimes referred to as *informative*).

To explain the distinction between these three types it is necessary to introduce a little nomenclature:

- For each patient it is planned to make a sequence of T observations, $Y_1, Y_2, \ldots, Y_T$. In addition, for each patient there may be a set of fixed covariates, X, assumed fully observed.
- Missing values arise from individuals dropping out, so that if Y_k is missing, then so also are $Y_{k+1}, \ldots, Y_T$.
- Define a drop-out indicator D for each patient, where $D = k$ if the patient drops out between the $(k-1)$th and kth observation time, and $D = T + 1$ if the patient does not drop out.

Completely random drop-out (MCAR) occurs when patients drop out of the study in a process which is independent of both the observed measurements and those that would have been available had they not been missing, so that

$$\Pr(D = k | X, Y_1, \ldots, Y_T) = \Pr(D = k) \qquad (3.1)$$

Here the observed (non-missing) values effectively constitute a simple random sample of the values for all study subjects. Examples include missing laboratory measurements because of a dropped test-tube (if it was not dropped because of the knowledge of any measurement), the accidental death of a participant in a study, or a participant moving to another area. Intermittent missing values in a longitudinal data set might also often reasonably be assumed to be MCAR, though supporting evidence would usually be required. Completely random drop-out causes least problem for data analysis, but it is a strong assumption.

Little (1995) distinguishes completely random dropout from *covariate-dependent* dropout, for which

$$\Pr(D = k \,|\, X, Y_1, \ldots, Y_T) = \Pr(D = k \,|\, X) \tag{3.2}$$

and the probability of dropping out depends on the values of the fixed covariates X, but given X, it is conditionally independent of an individual's outcome values, $Y_1, \ldots, Y_T$. Such a definition allows dependence of drop-out on both between-subject and within-subject covariates that can be treated as fixed in the model. In particular, if X includes, for example, a treatment group indicator or gender, this definition allows the drop-out rates to vary over treatment groups or between men and women. This can be illustrated in a non-medical context by a survey in which females are less likely to provide their personal income in general, independent of their actual income. If the sex of every individual is known, and we have income levels for some of the women, unbiased, sex-specific income estimates can be made, since the incomes we do have of these women are a random sample of all female incomes.

With completely random drop-out it is not necessary to construct a model for the drop-out mechanism or the missing observations, although in any model for the observed values it is important to include covariates that are predictive of drop-out.

The MAR mechanism occurs when the drop-out process depends on the outcome measures that have been observed in the past, but given that this information is conditionally independent of all the future (unrecorded) values of the outcome variable following drop-out, so that

$$\Pr(D = k \,|\, X, Y_1, \ldots, Y_T) = \Pr(D = k \,|\, X, Y_1, \ldots, Y_{k-1}) \tag{3.3}$$

Here 'missingness' depends only on the observed data, with the distribution of future values for a subject who drops out at time t being the same as the distribution of the future values of a subject who remains in at time t, if they have the same covariates and the same past history of outcome up to and including time t.

Murray and Findlay (1988) provide an example of this type of missing value from a study of hypertensive drugs in which the outcome measure was diastolic blood pressure. The protocol of the study specified that the participant was to be removed from the study when his/her blood pressure became too high. Here blood pressure at the time of drop-out was observed before the participant dropped out, so although the missing value mechanism is not MCAR since it depends on the values of blood pressure, it *is* MAR, because drop-out depends only on the observed part of Y.

The final type of missing-data mechanism is that known as non-ignorable or informative, in which missingness depends on the unrecorded missing values – observations are likely to be missing when the true values are systematically higher or lower. A non-medical example is when individuals with lower income levels or very high incomes are less likely to provide their personal income in an interview. In a medical setting possible examples are a participant dropping out of a longitudinal study when his/her blood pressure became too high and this value was not observed, or when their pain become intolerable and the associated pain value was not recorded. Dealing with data containing missing values of this type can be difficult.

Before we move on to discuss the implications of this taxonomy of missing values for the analysis of studies in which such values occur, we need to briefly consider how we can decide which type of missing-data mechanism applies to a particular data set. Unfortunately there is no completely satisfactory answer to this question, but there are a number of relatively simple and largely informal procedures that may be helpful in specific cases.

The first of these procedures is graphical and was first suggested by Diggle (1998). Participants in the trial are divided retrospectively into cohorts, according to their drop-out times, and a plot is made of the observed mean response as a function of time within each of the resulting groups, ignoring treatments. Diggle provides an example of this type of plot using data from a trial comparing drug regimes in the treatment of chronic schizophrenia. Six treatments were involved (coded p = placebo, h = haloperidol 20 mg, $r2$ = risperidone 2 mg, $r6$ = risperidone 6 mg, $r10$ = risperidone 10 mg, $r16$ = risperidone 16 mg) and the numbers of drop-outs and completers by treatment group were as follows:

	p	h	r2	r6	r10	r16	Total
Drop-outs	61	51	51	34	39	34	270
Completers	27	36	36	52	48	54	253
Total	88	87	87	86	87	88	523

The response variable in the study was a measure of psychiatric disorder, higher values indicating more severe illness. The observed mean responses for all six treatment groups are shown in Figure 3.1. There is a general decline in the response over time. The plot of the response profiles of each of the dropout cohorts is shown in Figure 3.2. The mean response for completers is qualitatively similar to all the profiles in Figure 3.1, except for a steeper initial decrease and a levelling out towards the end of the study. Within each of the other drop-out cohorts, however, the picture is quite different. In each of these the mean score increases immediately prior to drop-out. Clearly it would not be reasonable to analyse these data using any methods that assumed the missing values to be MCAR, since dropping out is clearly related to the values of the response variable.

Another possibility for investigating the drop-out mechanism is to apply a logistic regression to the probability of dropping out at a particular time, using, for example, the previous time's response value as an explanatory variable. Applying this method to the pain data in Table 3.1 shows that the previous response value *is* predictive of dropping out. The estimated regression coefficient is 0.009 with a standard error of 0.004. The drop in deviance from the null model is 4.53. So dropping out in these data is dependent on the value of the response. A plot of pain score against predicted probability of dropping out found from the logistic regression, shown in Figure 3.3, makes this relationship very clear.

Other procedures for assessing the drop-out mechanism are described in Carpenter *et al.* (2002).

3.2.2 Complete-case analysis

At one time a frequently used method for dealing with longitudinal data containing missing values, complete-case analysis is now no longer regarded as respectable by statisticians. The reasons are not difficult to identify. Complete-case analysis only

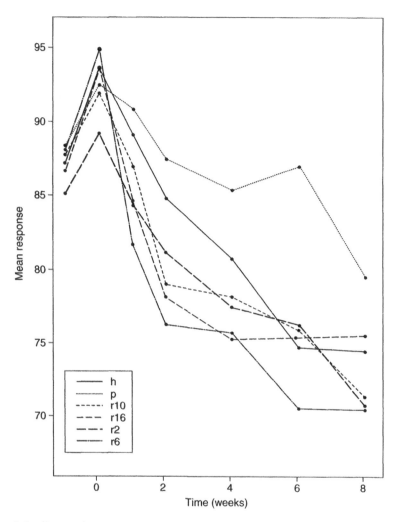

Figure 3.1 Observed mean response profiles for the schizophrenia trial data. (Taken with permission from Diggle, 1998.)

gives valid inferences when the missing values are MCAR, since then the complete cases are a random subsample of the original sample with respect to all variables. Even when the MCAR assumption is true, however, complete-case analysis remains objectionable because the rejection of incomplete cases is an unnecessary waste of information that reduces the effective sample size, and makes any modelling and associated estimation process inefficient and suboptimal.

But inefficiency may be a relatively minor problem of complete-case analysis compared to the difficulties that arise when the missing data are *not* MCAR. In such cases (which are likely to be the majority), the complete cases are often a biased sample, with the size of the resulting bias depending on the degree of deviation from MCAR, the amount of missing data, and the specifics of the analysis.

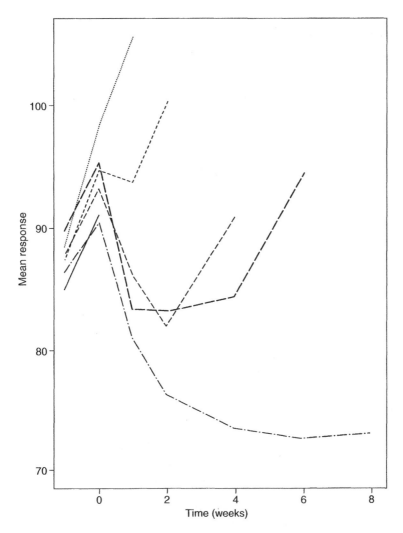

Figure 3.2 Observed mean response profiles for the schizophrenia trial data within each dropout cohort, ignoring treatments. (Taken with permission from Diggle, 1998.)

Because of these problems, complete-case analysis should now no longer be applied to longitudinal data with missing values; it is unnecessary since other more suitable alternatives are now readily available, as we shall describe in the following two subsections.

3.2.3 Imputation

According to Schafer (1999):

> Imputation, the practice of 'filling in' missing data with plausible values, has long been recognized as an attractive approach to analysing incomplete

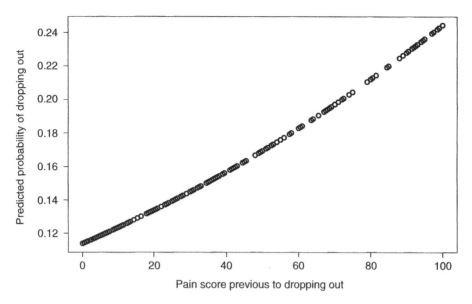

Figure 3.3   Predicted probability of dropping out for the pain data in Table 3.1 against previous response value.

> data … From an operational stand point, imputation solves the missing-data problem at the outset, enabling the analyst to proceed without further hindrance.

Certainly methods that impute missing values have the advantage that, unlike complete-case analysis, observed values in the incomplete cases are retained. But some imputation methods can create more problems than they solve, possibly distorting parameter estimates, standard errors and hypothesis tests, so careful consideration is needed of which method to use. For example, a simple, and still commonly used, method imputes missing values by their sample marginal means, perhaps calculated within a participant's own treatment group. In the pain data in Table 3.1, for example, we might replace the missing values in each group by the appropriate mean value chosen from the following observed means, calculated from the recorded pain values:

	30	60	90	120	150	180
Active	16.34	17.91	16.38	18.20	21.12	28.34
Placebo	27.47	37.00	47.12	65.59	75.55	77.63

But the only thing in favour of using this *unconditional mean* approach would be its simplicity. Even if the data are MCAR, which is unlikely, this type of imputation will lead to confidence intervals and inferences which may be seriously distorted by bias and overstated precision (variances will clearly be underestimated, since the imputed cases contribute zero to the sum of squared deviations from sample means).

Another simple, and also widely used, imputation method is to replace the missing values due to a participant dropping out with that participant's last observed value.

Table 3.3   Results of fitting an independence model to unconditional mean and LOCF imputed data sets

(a) Unconditional mean

Covariate	Estimated regression coefficient	Standard error	z-value
Intercept	−2.586	2.834	−0.913
Group	35.353	2.291	15.434
Time	0.212	0.022	9.504

(Dispersion parameter for Gaussian family taken to be 652.)
Null deviance: 537 284 on 497 degrees of freedom.
Residual deviance: 322 950 on 495 degrees of freedom.

(b) LOCF

Covariate	Estimated regression coefficient	Standard error	z-value
Intercept	3.520	3.509	1.00
Group	28.523	2.837	10.055
Time	0.155	0.028	5.611

(Dispersion parameter for Gaussian family taken to be 1000.)
Null deviance: 627 894 on 497 degrees of freedom.
Residual deviance: 495 242 on 495 degrees of freedom.

This is usually referred to as the *last observation carried forward* (LOCF) procedure. Clearly, this method makes a very strong assumption about the missing data, namely that the missing values on a case are all identical to the last observed value. Again this approach is likely to lead to a systematic underestimation of variability and is not recommended.

To illustrate the use of simple imputation we shall apply both the unconditional mean and LOCF procedures to the labour pain data, and then analyse the 'complete' data set using a regression model in which the repeated observations are assumed to be independent of one another. The data could, of course, be analysed under more realistic assumptions about the correlational structure of the repeated measurements, but we leave this as an exercise for the reader (see Exercise 3.2).

The results of fitting a regression model to each 'complete' data set, using treatment group and time as covariates, are shown in Table 3.3 The two simple methods of filling in the missing values lead, for these data, to exactly the same conclusion, namely that there is a large treatment effect and a substantial time effect.

But both unconditional mean and LOCF imputation cannot be recommended for general use for the reasons given above. More appropriate is some form of *multiple imputation*. This is a technique in which the missing values are replaced by more than one set of imputed values, usually between three and ten. Each of the 'complete' data sets is analysed by standard methods and the results are later combined to produce estimates and confidence intervals that incorporate missing-data uncertainty. In modern computing environments, the effort needed to produce and analyse a multiple-imputed data set is often not substantially greater than that required for single imputation. The multiply imputed data sets usually arise from *Bayesian models*, full details of which are given in Schafer (1999). One such method is based on what are known as *propensity scores*, and proceeds as follows:

- Carry out a logistic regression of the missing-value indicator of each observation on selected covariates.
- To each case assign a propensity score equal to $\mathbf{x}_i'\hat{\boldsymbol{\beta}}$, where $\hat{\boldsymbol{\beta}}$ is the vector of estimated regression coefficients from the step above, and $\mathbf{x}_i'$ is the vector of covariate values for individual i.
- For each missing value of the response variable construct a subset of observed response values from observations that have propensity scores 'close' to the score of the missing observation – this is known as the *donor pool*. ('Close' can be defined in a variety of ways; for example, we could take the 20 closest matches.)
- For each missing value, the imputations are generated from its donor pool according to an approximate Bayesian bootstrap method, described in Schafer (1999).

For the pain data, the score at the 30 min measurement occasion was used as the single covariate, with imputation being undertaken separately within each treatment group. Five imputed data sets were considered, and each analysed using the same model as used in the unconditional mean and LOCF imputation example above, that is, one including group and time as explanatory variables and assuming the repeated measurements were independent. The estimated parameters corresponding to each imputed data set are shown in Table 3.4.

Table 3.4   Results of fitting an independence model to five multiply imputed data sets

Data set 1

Covariate	Estimated regression coefficient	Standard error	Estimate/SE
Intercept	−4.472	3.217	−1.390
Group	33.431	2.600	12.860
Time	0.266	0.025	10.490

(Dispersion parameter for Gaussian family taken to be 840.6.)
Null deviance: 647 584 on 497 degrees of freedom.
Residual deviance: 416 094 on 495 degrees of freedom.

Data set 2

Covariate	Estimated regression coefficient	Standard error	Estimate/SE
Intercept	−5.982	3.315	−1.805
Group	36.200	2.680	13.509
Time	0.270	0.026	10.343

(Dispersion parameter for Gaussian family taken to be 892.)
Null deviance: 700 360 on 497 degrees of freedom.
Residual deviance: 441 923 on 495 degrees of freedom.

(Continued)

Table 3.4   (*Continued*)

Data set 3

Covariate	Estimated regression coefficient	Standard error	Estimate/SE
Intercept	−4.916	3.309	−1.486
Group	34.862	2.675	13.03
Time	0.257	0.026	9.847

(Dispersion parameter for Gaussian family taken to be 889.)
Null deviance: 677 754 on 497 degrees of freedom.
Residual deviance: 440 374 on 495 degrees of freedom.

Data set 4

Covariate	Estimated regression coefficient	Standard error	Estimate/SE
Intercept	−4.215	3.354	−1.257
Group	33.883	2.711	12.500
Time	0.260	0.026	9.849

(Dispersion parameter for Gaussian family taken to be 913.)
Null deviance: 683 614 on 497 degrees of freedom.
Residual deviance: 452 248 on 495 degrees of freedom.

Data set 5

Covariate	Estimated regression coefficient	Standard error	Estimate/SE
Intercept	−4.595	3.364	−1.366
Group	34.096	2.719	12.538
Time	0.263	0.027	9.911

(Dispersion parameter for Gaussian family taken to be 919.)
Null deviance: 690 038 on 497 degrees of freedom.
Residual deviance: 455 176 on 495 degrees of freedom.

The combined estimate of any of the regression coefficients is simply the average of the five separate values; for treatment group, for example, this gives a value of 34.49. Calculating the pooled standard error (PSE) of the regression coefficient is a little more tricky. The appropriate formula is

$$\text{PSE} = \sqrt{\text{ASE} + (1 + 1/m)\text{BSE}} \tag{3.4}$$

where m is the number of data sets constructed, ASE is the average of the variances of the parameter from each imputed data set and BSE is the between-imputation variance, given by

$$\text{BSE} = \frac{1}{m-1}\sum_{i=1}^{m}(\text{parameter estimate for data set } i - \text{average parameter value})^2$$

$$\tag{3.5}$$

For treatment group this results in BSE = 1.178, and ASE is 7.168, leading to a value for PSE of 2.881.

The conclusions to be drawn from this more complex analysis are, for this particular data set in which the treatment and time effects are both very large, the same as those arrived at by using the simpler imputation methods. But this will not always be the case, particularly when the effects of covariates are more subtle. Multiple imputation is the preferred option, particularly since it can now be applied routinely using the software listed at the end of the chapter.

3.3   Modelling longitudinal data containing ignorable missing values

Complete-case analysis and imputation both result in a rectangular data matrix to analyse. At one time this was an important consideration since the methods (and software) used to deal with longitudinal data could only cope with situations in which each individual in the study had the same number of repeated measurements of the response, taken at the same time points. But as we have already indicated in Chapter 2, this is no longer a requirement for current modelling techniques applicable to longitudinal data. Consequently, any of the methods described in Chapter 2 could be applied to a data set such as that in Table 3.1 after reorganization into the 'long' form in which each individual contributes as many records as repeated measures. Arranged in this way, missing values can now be ignored in any analysis, without the available observations for an individual being excluded.

A question that needs to be asked, however, is under what type of missing-data mechanism the various methods are valid. Let us begin by considering the question in the context of responses which can be assumed to follow a Gaussian distribution, and for which maximum likelihood estimation is possible.

For likelihood-based inference, the critical distinction is between MCAR and MAR (often referred to collectively as *ignorable*) and informative drop-out, since in the former case the log-likelihood function used as the basis of estimation is separable into two terms, one involving the missing-data mechanism given the observed values and one only the observed values. The first of these contains no information about the distribution of observed values and can therefore be ignored for the purposes of making inferences about these values. (Details of the mathematics behind this argument can be found in Diggle *et al.*, 1994.) Consequently, the models considered in Chapter 2 for Gaussian responses are applicable to data containing missing values under the less stringent requirement that these are MAR, rather than the strong MCAR assumption. What happens when the missing values are non-ignorable, and under what conditions the generalized estimating equations approach is valid, will be taken up after considering some further analyses of the pain data.

3.3.1   Modelling the pain data

Part of the pain data in Table 3.1, rearranged into the long form, is shown in Table 3.5. Here we shall consider two relatively simple random effects models for the data, one that includes only a random intercept and one that includes both a random intercept and a random slope effect for time. The results of fitting both models are shown in Table 3.6.

Table 3.5 Part of the pain data in
Table 3.1 rearranged into long form

Subject	Time	Pain score
1	30	0.0
1	60	0.0
1	90	0.0
1	120	NA
1	150	NA
1	180	NA
2	30	0.0
2	60	0.0
2	90	0.0
2	120	2.5
2	150	2.3
2	180	14.0

Table 3.6 Results of fitting two random effects models to the pain data

Random intercept

Covariate	Estimated regression coefficient	Standard error	Estimate/SE
Intercept	0.400	4.370	0.091
Group	28.141	5.740	4.902
Time	0.228	0.022	10.364

$\hat{\sigma}_u = 24.09$, $\hat{\sigma} = 18.6$.

Random intercept and slope

Covariate	Estimated regression coefficient	Standard error	Estimate/SE
Intercept	1.673	4.936	0.339
Group	25.162	5.783	4.351
Time	0.225	0.039	5.778

$\hat{\sigma}_{u_1} = 34.081$, $\hat{\sigma}_{u_2} = 0.293$, $\hat{\rho}_{u_1 u_2} = -0.683$, $\hat{\sigma} = 12.464$.

Comparison of the two models

	Model	df	Log-likelihood	Test	Likelihood ratio	p-value
Random intercept	1	7	−1585			
Random intercept and slope	2	5	−1635	1 vs 2	100.9	<0.0001

The results show that the random intercept and slope model provides a better description of these data, although the conclusions to be drawn from fitting either model are the same, a large treatment effect and a large time effect. The active treatment reduces the average pain score by between about 17 and 40 points, and pain

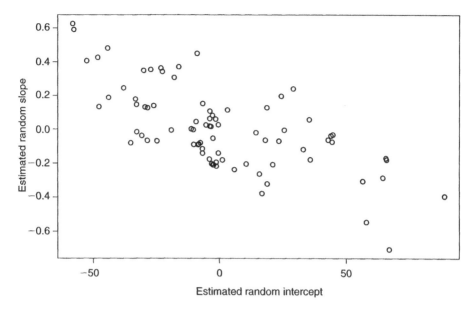

Figure 3.4 Plot of estimated slope against estimated intercept for pain data.

increases with time. The estimated correlation between the slope and random intercept effects in the second model is -0.68. Larger intercepts appear to be associated with smaller slopes, and vice versa (see Figure 3.4). This large negative correlation arises because all the data were collected between times 30 and 180 min, but the intercept represents the measurement at time zero. The correlation can be removed by centring the data, that is, by using time minus its mean value as covariate rather than time itself. Since the results of most interest, in particular the estimate of the treatment effect, remain unchanged when fitting the new model, this is left as an exercise for the reader.

For non-Gaussian responses, for example a binary variable, the generalized estimating equation approach was introduced in Chapter 2. This is a quasi-likelihood (rather than a likelihood proper) method, so the question about when the approach is valid is not answered by the comments made about the log-likelihood function mentioned at the beginning of this section. In fact the GEE method is only valid when the missing-data mechanism is MCAR. When the data are not MCAR then the estimates produced by GEE are biased, although Robins *et al.* (1995) show how to introduce weights to allow for the pattern of missingness which, if used, allow the method to be valid under the weaker MAR assumption. An example is given in Everitt and Pickles (2000).

3.4 Non-ignorable missing values

Informative missing values are both difficult to deal with and, in most cases, impossible to detect from the observed data. But both likelihood and GEE methods are biased when there is non-ignorable missingness, and so a number of authors have considered the difficult problem of how to analyse longitudinal data if the missing values *are* informative. Diggle and Kenward (1994), for example, propose a modelling framework for this situation, in which random or completely random drop-outs are included as explicit models. But the essential feature is a logistic model for the probability of dropping out, in which the explanatory variables can include previous values of the response variable, but in addition can include the unobserved value at drop-out as a latent variable. In other words, the drop-out probability can be allowed to depend on both the observed measurement history and the unobserved value at drop-out. Software for fitting the model is available (details are given at the end of the chapter), and examples of its use are given in Diggle *et al.* (1994) and Everitt and Pickles (2000).

The Diggle–Kenward model represents a welcome addition to the methodology available for analysing longitudinal data in which there are drop-outs. But as with any new modelling framework, questions need to be asked about its adequacy in practical situations. Matthews (1994), for example, makes the point that if there are many drop-outs, the proposed model *can* be applied, but questions whether many statisticians would feel happy to rely on technical virtuosity when 60% of the data are absent. Alternatively, if the proportion of drop-outs is low, then much less can be learnt about the drop-out process, leading to low power to discriminate between drop-out processes. Skinner (1994) suggests that the longitudinal data remaining after drop-out may, by themselves, contain very little information about the 'informativeness' of the drop-out and concludes that external information about the drop-out mechanism be sought and used. A further possible problem identified by Troxel *et al.* (1998) is that the bias that results from assuming the wrong type of missingness mechanism may well be more severe than the bias that results from misspecification of a standard full maximum likelihood model.

Despite these and other reservations made in the discussion of Diggle and Kenward's paper, their proposed model does open up the possibility of some further investigation of the drop-out process. An interesting recent example of the application of their methodology is given in Carpenter *et al.* (2002).

3.5 Compliance and intention-to-treat

Although our main concern in this chapter has been to illustrate how to analyse appropriately data from longitudinal studies in which missing values occur, there are two important related issues which it is also convenient to discuss here: *compliance* and *intention-to-treat*.

Compliance means participants following both the intervention regimen and trial procedures – for example, clinic visits, laboratory procedures and filling out forms. In particular, participants continue to comply with the treatment to which they were randomly assigned. In an ideal trial all participants would comply in this way, but in reality, things are often far from ideal, for reasons succinctly outlined by Efron (1998).

> There could be no worse experimental animals on earth than human beings: they complain, they go on vacations, they take things they are not supposed to take, they live incredibly complicated lives, and, sometimes, they do not take their medicine.

In many clinical trials participants frequently fail to adhere to the treatment to which they were originally assigned. Poor participant compliance can adversely affect the outcome of a trial so it is important to use methods both to improve and monitor level of compliance. Level of compliance will depend on a number of factors, including:

- the amount of time and inconvenience involved in making follow-up visits to the clinic;
- the perceived importance of the procedures performed at each visit from a health maintenance point of view;
- the potential health benefits associated with treatment versus potential risks;
- the amount of discomfort produced by the study treatments or procedures performed;
- the amount of effort required of the patient to maintain the treatment regime;
- the number and type of side-effects associated with treatment.

In recent times the problems of non-compliance in a clinical trial have been well illustrated in trials involving HIV/AIDS patients, where an atmosphere of rapidly alternating hopes and disappointments has added to the difficulties of keeping patients on a fixed long-term treatment schedule. So what can be done to ensure maximum patient compliance? Aspects of the study design may help; the shorter the trial, for example, the more likely subjects are to comply with the intervention regimen. So a study started and completed in one day would have great advantages over longer trials. And studies in which the subjects are under close supervision, such as in-patient hospital-based trials, tend to have fewer problems of non-compliance.

Simplicity of intervention may also affect compliance, with single-dose drug regimens usually being preferable to those requiring multiple doses. The interval between scheduled visits to hospital or clinic is also a factor to consider. Too long an interval between visits may lead to a steady fall in patient compliance due to lack of encouragement, while too short an interval may prove a nuisance and reduce cooperation.

Perhaps the most important factor in maintaining good subject compliance once a trial has begun is the attitude of the staff running the trial. Experienced investigators stay in close contact with the patients early after randomization to get patients involved and, later, to keep them interested when their initial enthusiasm may have worn off. On the other hand, uninterested or discourteous staff will lead to an uninterested patient population. Meinert (1986) lists a number of simple factors likely to enhance patient participation and interest; this list is reproduced in Table 3.7.

One widely used method for improving compliance is the use of a *placebo run-in*, in which potential participants in a trial are asked to take placebo pills for a short period of time (they are not told they are placebos). If the participant takes the pills as instructed, then she is entered into the trial. However, if the participant does not comply with the instructions on pill taking, then she is excluded from the trial. The assumption underlying the placebo run-in is that participants who do not comply in short term run-ins are more likely not to comply with long-term therapy; Dari *et al.* (1995) and Trivedi and Rush (1994) have challenged this assumption.

Monitoring compliance is a crucial part of many clinical trials, since according to Friedman *et al.* (1985):

> the interpretation of study results will be influenced by knowledge of compliance with the intervention. To the extent that the control group is not truly a control group and the intervention group is not being treated as intended, group differences may be diluted, leading possibly to an underestimate of the therapeutic effect and an underreporting of adverse effects.

Table 3.7 Factors and approaches that enhance patient interest and participation

---

- Clinic staff who treat patients with courtesy and dignity and who take an interest in meeting their needs.
- Clinic located in pleasant physical surroundings and in a secure environment.
- Convenient access to parking for patients who drive, and to other modes of transportation for those who do not.
- Payment of parking and travel fees incurred by study patients.
- Payment of clinic registration fees and costs for procedures required in the trial.
- Special clinics in which patients are able to avoid the confusion and turmoil of a regular out-patient clinic.
- Scheduled appointments designed to minimize waiting time.
- Clinic hours designed for patient convenience.
- Written or telephone contacts between clinic visits.
- Remembering patients on special occasions, such as Christmas, birthdays, anniversaries, etc.
- Establishment of identity with the study through proper indoctrination and explanation of study procedures during the enrolment process; through procedures such as the use of special ID cards to identify the patient as a participant in the study, and by awarding certificates to recognize their contributions to the trial.

Source: Meinert (1986).

Feinstein (1991) points out that differential compliance to two equally effective regimens can also lead to possibly erroneous conclusions about the effect of the intervention.

In some studies measuring compliance is relatively easy – for example, trials in which one group receives surgery and the other group does not. Most of the time, however, assessment of compliance is not so simple and can rarely be established perfectly. In drug trials one of the most commonly used methods of evaluating subject compliance is pill or capsule count. But the method is far from foolproof. Even when a subject returns the appropriate number of leftover pills at a scheduled visit, the question of whether the remaining pills were used according to the protocol remains largely unanswered. Good rapport with the subjects will encourage cooperation and lead to a more accurate pill count, although there is considerable evidence that shows that the method can be unreliable and potentially misleading (see Cramer *et al.*, 1988; Waterhouse *et al.*, 1993).

Laboratory determinations can also sometimes be used to monitor compliance with medications. Tests done on either blood or urine can detect the presence of active drugs or metabolites. For example, Hjalmarson *et al.* (1981) checked compliance with metroprobol therapy after myocardial infarction by using assays of metroprobol in urine. Several other approaches to monitoring compliance are described in Friedman *et al.* (1985), and Senn (1997) mentions two recent technical developments that may be useful, namely:

- electronic monitoring – pill dispensers with a built-in microchip which will log when the dispenser was opened;
- low-dose, slow-turnover chemical markers that can be added to treatment and then detected via blood-sampling.

The claim is often made that in published drug trials more than 90% of patients have been satisfactorily compliant with the protocol-specified dosing regimen. But Urquhart and de Klerk (1998) suggest that these claims are exaggerated, based as they usually are on count of returned dosing forms, which patients can easily manipulate, and that data from the more reliable methods for measuring compliance, mentioned above, contradict them.

Non-compliance may lead to the investigator transferring a patient to the alternative therapy or withdrawing the patient from the study altogether; often such decisions are taken out of the investigator's hands by the patient simply refusing to participate in the trial any further and thus becoming a trial drop-out. When non-compliance manifests as drop-out from a study, the connection with missing data is direct. In other circumstances manifestation of non-compliance is more complex and some response is observed, but a question remains about what would have been observed had compliance been achieved.

Non-compliance, leading either to receiving treatment other than that provided for by the results of randomization, or to dropping out of the trial altogether, has serious implications for the analysis of the data collected in a clinical trial. The drop-out problem has been dealt with earlier in the chapter, but what about the possible lack of adherence to treatment?

In most randomized clinical trials not all patients adhere to the therapy to which they were randomly assigned. Instead they may receive the therapy assigned to another treatment group, or even a therapy different from any prescribed in the protocol. When such non-adherence occurs, problems arise with the analysis comparing the treatments under study. There are a number of possibilities, of which the following are the most common:

- *intention-to-treat* or *analysis-as-randomized*, in which analysis is based on original treatment assignment rather than treatment actually received;
- *adherers-only method*, that is, analysing only those patients who adhered to the original treatment assignment;
- *treatment-received method*, that is, analysing patients according to the treatment ultimately received.

The intention-to-treat approach requires that any comparison of the treatments is based upon comparison of the outcome results of all patients in the treatment groups to which they were randomly assigned. This approach is recommended since it maintains the benefits of randomization, whereas the adherers-only and treatment-received methods compare groups that have *not* been randomized to their respective treatments; consequently, the analyses may be subject to unknown biases and for this reason most statisticians and drug regulatory agencies prefer intention-to-treat. But although it is clear that analyses based on compliance are inherently biased because non-compliance does not occur randomly, many clinicians (and even some statisticians) have criticized analysis that does not reflect the treatment actually received, especially when many patients do not remain on the initially assigned therapy (see, for example, Feinstein, 1991). In the face of substantial non-compliance, it is not difficult to understand the intuitive appeal of comparing only those patients in the original trial who actually complied with the prescribed treatment. However, in addition to the difficulty of defining compliance in an objective manner, subjects who comply tend to fare differently and in a somewhat unpredictable way from those who do not comply. Thus any observed difference among treatment groups constructed in this way may be due not to treatment but to factors associated with compliance.

The target of estimation implicit in an intention-to-treat analysis has been called the *pragmatic effectiveness*, which combines the average therapeutic effect of the treatment and the rate of patient compliance to the treatment regimen. Dissatisfaction with this approach usually reflects the desire of the investigator to estimate the *biologic efficacy* of the treatment regardless of compliance. But none of the three methods of analysis mentioned above can get at this without using compliance information, and attempts to do this can lead to substantial selection bias.

An interesting illustration of the different conclusions that can result from using the three methods is given by Peduzzi *et al.* (1993), who compare the methods on simulated data for a hypothetical cohort of 350 medical and 350 surgical patients having exponentially distributed survival times and assuming a 10-year survival rate of 50% in each group. In addition, they generated an independent exponential time to 'cross-over' for each of the 350 medical patients, assuming half the patients crossed over by 10 years. Medical cross-overs were then defined as those patients with time to cross-over less than survival time. Figure 3.5 displays 10-year survival rates by the as-randomized, adherers-only, and treatment-received methods. The latter two methods demonstrate a consistent survival advantage in favour of surgical therapy, when by definition there is actually no difference in survival between the two treatment groups.

According to Efron (1998):

> Statistics deals with the analysis of complicated noisy phenomena, never more so than in its applications to biomedical research, and in this noisy world the intent-to-treat analysis of a randomised double-blinded clinical trial stands as a flagpole of certainty amongst the chaos.

Indeed, according to Goetghebeur and Shapiro (1996), intention-to-treat analysis has achieved the status of a 'best unbiased inference with regard to causal knowledge' or BUICK. Many statisticians would endorse these views and also find themselves largely in agreement with Peduzzi *et al.* (1993):

> We conclude that the method of analysis should be consistent with the experimental design of a study. For randomised trials, such consistency requires the preservation of the random treatment assignment. Because methods that violate the principles of randomisation are susceptible to bias, we are against their use.

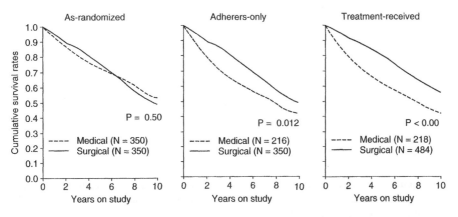

Figure 3.5 Ten-year survival rates by the as-randomized, adherers-only and treatment-received approaches for a set of simulated data. (Taken with permission from Peduzzi *et al.*, 1993, by permission of the publisher, John Wiley and Sons, Ltd.)

3.6　Summary

Missing values caused by participants dropping out are a fact of life in most longitudinal studies undertaken in medicine. Trying to decide whether such values are MCAR, MAR or informative is an important but often difficult aspect of the analysis of the data that result. Various relatively informal methods discussed in this chapter can be helpful, but often no definite decision can be made. In many cases modelling techniques that assume only MAR are likely to give reasonable results. Imputing missing values is a possible alternative, but care needs to be taken to use an appropriate technique, such as multiple imputation.

Software

Software for multiple imputation is available but is more restricted than that described for the techniques in Chapters 1 and 2. Examples of relevant procedures are:

SAS　　　`proc mi` (multiple imputation);
　　　　　`proc mianalyze` (combines results of the multiple imputation).

S-PLUS　A comprehensive missing-data library is available in S-PLUS 6; features of the library are described in the excellent accompanying on-line manual (see Schimert *et al.*, 2000). The library is attached using `library(missing)`.

SOLAS　A package marketed by Statistical Solutions Ltd, 8 South Bank, Crosse's Green, Cork, Ireland, which allows both single imputation and multiple imputation by a variety of the methods described in Chapter 3. Includes facilities for combining statistics for imputed data sets.

Software for multiple imputation is reviewed in Horton and Lipsitz (2000).

OSWALD　The Diggle–Kenward method for handling dropouts is implemented in this software (Object oriented Software for the Analysis of Longitudinal Data in S-PLUS) written by David Smith, Bill Robertson and Peter Diggle, and available from:
　　　　　http://www.maths.lancs.ac.uk/software/Oswald/

Exercises

3.1 For the pain data in Table 3.1, repeat the logistic regression for dropping out described in Section 3.2.1 but using treatment group as an additional covariate.

3.2 Calculate the combined results for the time regression coefficient in the multiply imputed data in Table 3.4.

3.3 Impute the pain data in Table 3.1 using both unconditional means and LOCF. To each imputed data set fit a random intercept model, and compare your results with those given in Section 3.3.

4

Generalized Additive Models

4.1 Introduction

The generalized linear model featured in Chapter 1 can accommodate nonlinear functions of the explanatory variables, for example quadratic or cubic terms, if these are thought to be necessary to provide an adequate fit (see Exercise 2.1). In this chapter, however, we consider some alternative (and generally more flexible) statistical methods for modelling nonlinear relationships between a response variable and one or more explanatory variables. The use of these methods, known as *generalized additive models* (GAMs), allows the fitting of a smooth relationship between two or more variables through a scatterplot of data points. GAMs are useful where

- the relationship between the variables is expected to be of complex form, not easily fitted by standard linear or nonlinear models;
- there is no a priori reason for using a particular model;
- we would like the data themselves to suggest the appropriate functional form.

Such models should be regarded as philosophically closer to the concepts of exploratory data analysis, in which the form of any functional relationship emerges from a set of data, rather than arising from a theoretical construct. In the health sciences, this can be especially useful because it reflects the uncertainty of knowledge regarding the mechanisms that determine disease and its prognosis.

The building blocks of the GAM approach are *scatterplot smoothers*, which are described in the next section.

4.2 Scatterplot smoothers

The scatterplot is an excellent first exploratory graph to study the dependence of two variables. An important second exploratory graph adds a smooth curve to the scatterplot to help us better perceive the pattern of dependence. Most readers will be familiar with adding a parametric curve, such as a simple linear or polynomial regression fit; however, there are nonparametric alternatives that are perhaps less familiar, but that can often be more useful, since many bivariate data sets are too complex to be described by a simple parametric family. Perhaps the simplest of these alternatives is a *locally weighted regression* or *loess* fit, first suggested by Cleveland (1979). In essence this approach assumes that the variables x and y are related by the equation

$$y_i = g(x_i) + \varepsilon_i \tag{4.1}$$

Table 4.1   Oxygen uptake and expired ventilation in 53 subjects

	Oxygen uptake	Expired ventilation		Oxygen uptake	Expired ventilation
1	574	21.9	28	2577	46.3
2	592	18.6	29	2766	55.8
3	664	18.6	30	2812	54.5
4	667	19.1	31	2893	63.5
5	718	19.2	32	2957	60.3
6	770	16.9	33	3052	64.8
7	927	18.3	34	3151	69.2
8	947	17.2	35	3161	74.7
9	1020	19.0	36	3266	72.9
10	1096	19.0	37	3386	80.4
11	1277	18.6	38	3452	83.0
12	1323	22.8	39	3521	86.0
13	1330	24.6	40	3543	88.9
14	1599	24.9	41	3676	96.8
15	1639	29.2	42	3741	89.1
16	1787	32.0	43	3844	100.9
17	1790	27.9	44	3878	103.0
18	1794	31.0	45	4002	113.4
19	1874	30.7	46	4114	111.4
20	2049	35.4	47	4152	119.9
21	2132	36.1	48	4252	127.2
22	2160	39.1	49	4290	126.4
23	2292	42.6	50	4331	135.5
24	2312	39.9	51	4332	138.9
25	2475	46.2	52	4390	143.7
26	2489	50.9	53	4393	144.8
27	2490	46.5			

where g is a 'smooth' function and the ε_i are random variables with mean zero and constant scale. Values $\hat{y}_i$ used to 'estimate' the y_i at each x_i are found by fitting polynomials using weighted least squares with large weights for points near to x_i and small weights otherwise. So smoothing takes place essentially by local averaging of the y-values of observations having predictor values close to a target value.

Two parameters control the shape of a loess curve. The first is a smoothing parameter, α, with larger values leading to smoother curves – typical values are from ¼ to 1. The second parameter, λ, is the degree of certain polynomials that are fitted by the method; λ can take value 1 or 2. In any specific application, the choice of the two parameters must be based on a combination of judgement and of trial and error. Residual plots may, however, be helpful in judging a particular combination of values.

We shall illustrate the use of locally weighted regression on the data shown in Table 4.1, which gives the oxygen uptake and the expired ventilation of a number of subjects performing a standard exercise task.

Figures 4.1(a)–(d) show plots of the data with added locally weighted regression fits with different values of λ and α. Here the four fitted curves are very similar, and, in this relatively simple case, each is almost identical to a fitted polynomial containing a quadratic term in oxygen uptake – see Figure 4.1(e).

A more difficult challenge for the locally weighted regression approach is provided by the data shown in Table 4.2; these are monthly deaths from bronchitis, emphysema and asthma in the UK from 1974 to 1979 for both men and women.

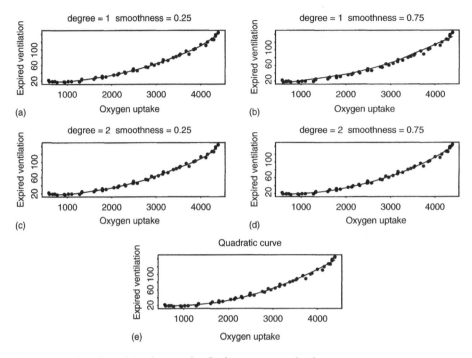

Figure 4.1   Locally weighted regression fits for oxygen uptake data.

Table 4.2   Monthly deaths from bronchitis, emphysema and asthma in the UK from 1974 to 1979 for both men and women

	Jan	Feb	Mar	Apr	May	Jun	Jul	Aug	Sep	Oct	Nov	Dec
1974	3035	2552	2704	2554	2014	1655	1721	1524	1596	2074	2199	2512
1975	2933	2889	2938	2497	1870	1726	1607	1545	1396	1787	2076	2837
1976	2787	3891	3179	2011	1636	1580	1489	1300	1356	1653	2013	2823
1977	2996	2523	2540	2520	1994	1964	1691	1479	1596	1877	2032	2484
1978	2899	2990	2890	2379	1933	1734	1617	1495	1440	1777	1970	2745
1979	2841	3535	3010	2091	1667	1589	1518	1348	1392	1619	1954	2633

Figure 4.2 shows a number of plots of the data with added locally weighted regression fits, again with different values of λ and α. Here the characteristic cyclical nature of the data is only picked up with $\lambda = 2$ and $\alpha = 0.25$. In the other three diagrams the amount of smoothing is too great to reveal the structure in the data.

An alternative smoother that can often usefully be applied to bivariate data is some form of *spline function*. (A spline is a term for a flexible strip of metal or rubber used by a draftsman to draw curves.) Spline functions are polynomials within intervals of the x-variable that are connected across different values of x. Figure 4.3, for example, shows a linear spline function, that is, a piecewise linear function, of the form

$$f(x) = \beta_0 + \beta_1 X + \beta_2 (X - a)_+ + \beta_3 (X - b)_+ + \beta_4 (X - c)_+ \qquad (4.2)$$

where

$$(u)_+ = \begin{cases} u & \text{if } u > 0 \\ 0 & \text{if } u \leq 0 \end{cases}$$

The interval endpoints, a, b, and c, are called *knots*. The number of knots can vary according to the amount of data available for fitting the function.

The linear spline is simple and can approximate some relationships, but it is not smooth and so will not fit highly curved functions well. The problem is overcome by using piecewise polynomials – in particular, cubics, which have been found to have

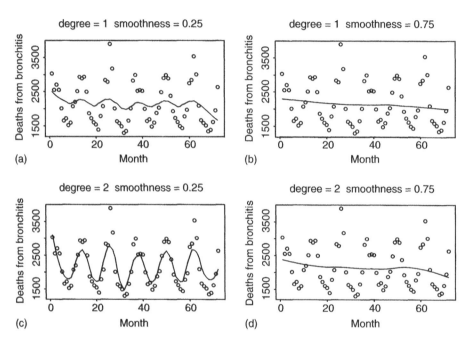

Figure 4.2   Locally weighted regression fits for the monthly deaths from bronchitis data.

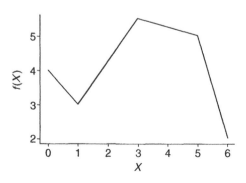

Figure 4.3   A linear spline function with knots at $a = 1$, $b = 3$, $c = 5$. (Taken from Harrell, 2001, with permission of the publisher, Springer-Verlag.)

nice properties with good ability to fit a variety of complex relationships. The result is a *cubic spline* which arises formally by seeking a smooth curve $g(x)$ to summarize the dependence of y on x, which minimizes the expression

$$\sum \left[y_i - g(x_i) \right]^2 + \lambda \int g''(x)^2 \, dx \qquad (4.3)$$

where $g''(x)$ represents the second derivative of $g(x)$ with respect to x. Although when written formally this criterion looks a little formidable, it is really nothing more than an effort to govern the trade-off between the goodness of fit of the data (as measured by $\sum [y_i - g(x_i)]^2$) and the 'wiggliness' or departure from linearity of g measured by $\int g''(x)^2 \, dx$; for a linear function, this part of (4.3) would be zero. The parameter λ governs the smoothness of g, with larger values resulting in a smoother curve. The cubic spline which minimizes (4.3) is a series of cubic polynomials joined at the unique observed values of the explanatory variable, x_i. (For more details, see Friedman, 1991).

The 'effective number of parameters' (analogous to the number of parameters in a parametric fit) or degrees of freedom of a cubic spline smoother is generally used to specify its smoothness rather than λ directly. A numerical search is then used to determine the value of λ corresponding to the required degrees of freedom. Roughly, the complexity of a cubic spline is about the same as a polynomial of degree one less than the degrees of freedom. But the cubic spline smoother 'spreads out' its parameters in a more even way and hence is much more flexible than is polynomial regression.

We can illustrate the use of cubic splines on the time series data in Table 4.2. Figure 4.4 shows a cubic spline fitted to the data; this indicates the structure in the observations very clearly.

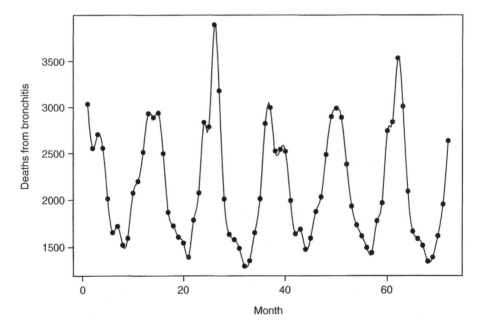

Figure 4.4 Cubic spline fit for the monthly deaths from bronchitis data.

4.3   Additive and generalized additive models

In a linear regression model there is a dependent variable, y, and a set of explanatory variables, $x_1, \ldots, x_q$, and the model assumed is

$$y = \beta_0 + \sum_{j=1}^{q} \beta_j x_j + \varepsilon \qquad (4.4)$$

Additive models replace the linear function $\beta_j x_j$ by a smooth nonparametric function to give

$$y = \beta_0 + \sum_{j=1}^{q} g_j(x_j) + \varepsilon \qquad (4.5)$$

where g_i can be one of the scatterplot smoothers described in the previous section, or, if the investigator chooses, a linear function for particular x_j. Models can therefore include a mixture of linear and smooth functions if necessary.

A GAM arises from (4.5) in the same way as a GLM arises from a multiple regression model, namely that some function of the expectation of the response variable is now modelled by a sum of nonparametric functions. So, for example, the logistic additive model is

$$\text{logit}[\Pr(y = 1)] = \beta_0 + \sum_{j=1}^{q} g_j(x_j) \qquad (4.6)$$

Fitting a GAM involves what is known as a *backfitting algorithm*. The smooth functions g_i are fitted one at a time by taking the residuals

$$y - \sum_{k \neq j} g_k(x_k) \qquad (4.7)$$

and fitting them against x_j using one of the scatterplot smoothers described in Section 4.2. The process is repeated until it converges. Linear terms in the model are fitted by least squares. Full details are given in Chambers and Hastie (1993).

Various tests are available to assess the nonlinear contributions of the fitted smoothers, and generalized additive models can be compared with, say, linear models fitted to the same data, by means of an F test on the residual sum of squares of the competing models. In this process the fitted smooth curve is assigned an estimated equivalent number of degrees of freedom. For full details again see Chambers and Hastie (1993).

4.4   Examples of the application of GAMs

Our first example will involve applying a GAM to the data shown in Table 4.3. These data are given in Hastie and Tibshirani (1990) and come from a study of the factors affecting patterns of insulin-dependent diabetes mellitus in children (Socket *et al.*, 1987). The objective was to investigate the dependence of the level of serum C-peptide on various other factors in order to understand the patterns of residual insulin secretion. The response measure to be used is the logarithm of C-peptide concentration at diagnosis, and the two explanatory variables are age and base deficit, a measure of acidity.

Table 4.3 Insulin-dependent diabetes in children

Subject	Age	Base deficit	Peptide	Subject	Age	Base deficit	Peptide
1	5.2	−8.1	4.8	23	11.3	−3.6	5.1
2	8.8	−16.1	4.1	24	1.0	−8.2	3.9
3	10.5	−0.9	5.2	25	14.5	−0.5	5.7
4	10.6	−7.8	5.5	26	11.9	−2.0	5.1
5	10.4	−29.0	5.0	27	8.1	−1.6	5.2
6	1.8	−19.2	3.4	28	13.8	−11.9	3.7
7	12.7	−18.9	3.4	29	15.5	−0.7	4.9
8	15.6	−10.6	4.9	30	9.8	−1.2	4.8
9	5.8	−2.8	5.6	31	11.0	−14.3	4.4
10	1.9	−25.0	3.7	32	12.4	−0.8	5.2
11	2.2	−3.1	3.9	33	11.1	−16.8	5.1
12	4.8	−7.8	4.5	34	5.1	−5.1	4.6
13	7.9	−13.9	4.8	35	4.8	−9.5	3.9
14	5.2	−4.5	4.9	36	4.2	−17.0	5.1
15	0.9	−11.6	3.0	37	6.9	−3.3	5.1
16	11.8	−2.1	4.6	38	13.2	−0.7	6.0
17	7.9	−2.0	4.8	39	9.9	−3.3	4.9
18	11.5	−9.0	5.5	40	12.5	−13.6	4.1
19	10.6	−11.2	4.5	41	13.2	−1.9	4.6
20	8.5	−0.2	5.3	42	8.9	−10.0	4.9
21	11.1	−6.1	4.7	43	10.8	−13.5	5.1
22	12.8	−1.0	6.6				

Source: Hastie and Tibshirani (1990).

Scatterplots of log(peptide) against age and against base are shown in Figure 4.5. Plotted on each of these are the associated linear regression and locally weighted regression fits. In both plots there appears to be at least some evidence of a departure from linearity, although this is stronger for age than for base deficit.

To begin, we fit a GAM to these data using locally weighted regression fits for both age and base (lo is used to denote a locally weighted fit). The results are shown in Table 4.4. The nonlinearity of age is confirmed, but it appears there is not a strong case for fitting a nonlinear term for base. A plot of the fitted functions is shown in Figure 4.6. Note the wide standard error limits for the base curve.

We now fit a model which includes a locally weighted regression fit for age but a linear term for base. A comparison of this model with the one described above (see Table 4.5) shows that allowing for possible nonlinearity of base contributes very little to the model.

Finally, we can compare the fit of the model with a locally weighted regression term for age and a linear term for base, with a multiple regression model which includes linear effects only for both explanatory variables: (again see Table 4.5). Allowing for nonlinearity in age contributes significantly to the model. We could, of course, allow for this nonlinearity in the classical way, by including, say, a quadratic term for age – we leave investigating this possibility as an exercise for the reader (see Exercise 4.1).

The next data set we shall consider is shown in Table 4.6. Again these data are given in Hastie and Tibshirani (1990); they involve observations on 81 children undergoing corrective surgery on the spine. There are a number of risk factors (explanatory variables) for *kyphosis*, or outward curvature of the spine in excess of 40 degrees from

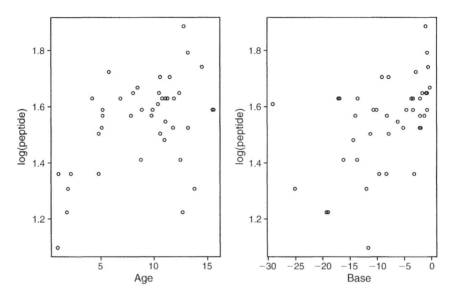

Figure 4.5 Scatterplots of log(peptide) against age and against base for insulin dependence data.

Table 4.4 Results of fitting a GAM model to insulin data in Table 4.3

	df npar.	df	npar. F	Pr(F)
Intercept	1			
lo(age)	1	3.3	4.689	0.006
lo(base)	1	3.0	2.065	0.124

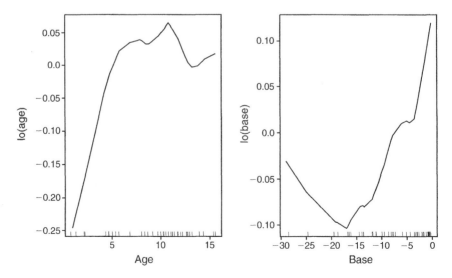

Figure 4.6 Fitted nonlinear functions for age and base.

Table 4.5   Results of fitting a GAM model to insulin dependent data

(a) Comparison of two GAM models

Model	Terms	Resid. df	Resid. dev.	Test	df	Deviance
1	lo(age) + base	36.72	0.4990			
2	lo(age) + lo(base)	33.73	0.4192	1 vs. 2	2.989	0.0798

(b) Comparison of GAM and multiple regression models

Model	Terms	Resid. df	RSS	Test	df	SS	F	Pr(F)
1	age + base	40	0.6685					
2	lo(age) + base	36.72	0.4990	1 vs. 2	3.278	0.1695	3.805	0.016

Table 4.6   Kyphosis data

	Kyphosis	Age (in months)	Number	Start		Kyphosis	Age (in months)	Number	Start
1	absent	71	3	5	35	absent	130	5	13
2	absent	158	3	14	36	absent	112	3	16
3	present	128	4	5	37	absent	140	5	11
4	absent	2	5	1	38	absent	93	3	16
5	absent	1	4	15	39	absent	1	3	9
6	absent	1	2	16	40	present	52	5	6
7	absent	61	2	17	41	absent	20	6	9
8	absent	37	3	16	42	present	91	5	12
9	absent	113	2	16	43	present	73	5	1
10	present	59	6	12	44	absent	35	3	13
11	present	82	5	14	45	absent	143	9	3
12	absent	148	3	16	46	absent	61	4	1
13	absent	18	5	2	47	absent	97	3	16
14	absent	1	4	12	48	present	139	3	10
16	absent	168	3	18	49	absent	136	4	15
17	absent	1	3	16	50	absent	131	5	13
18	absent	78	6	15	51	present	121	3	3
19	absent	175	5	13	52	absent	177	2	14
20	absent	80	5	16	53	absent	68	5	10
21	absent	27	4	9	54	absent	9	2	17
22	absent	22	2	16	55	present	139	10	6
23	present	105	6	5	56	absent	2	2	17
24	present	96	3	12	57	absent	140	4	15
25	absent	131	2	3	58	absent	72	5	15
26	present	15	7	2	59	absent	2	3	13
27	absent	9	5	13	60	present	120	5	8
29	absent	8	3	6	61	absent	51	7	9
30	absent	100	3	14	62	absent	102	3	13
31	absent	4	3	16	63	present	130	4	1
32	absent	151	2	16	64	present	114	7	8
33	absent	31	3	16	65	absent	81	4	1
34	absent	125	2	11	66	absent	118	3	16

(*Continued*)

Table 4.6   (*Continued*)

	Kyphosis	Age (in months)	Number	Start		Kyphosis	Age (in months)	Number	Start
67	absent	118	4	16	76	absent	206	4	10
68	absent	17	4	10	77	absent	11	3	15
69	absent	195	2	17	78	absent	178	4	15
70	absent	159	4	13	79	present	157	3	13
71	absent	18	4	11	80	absent	26	7	13
72	absent	15	5	16	81	absent	120	2	13
73	absent	158	5	14	82	present	42	7	6
74	absent	127	4	12	83	absent	36	4	13
75	absent	87	4	16					

Source: Hastie and Tibshirani (1990).

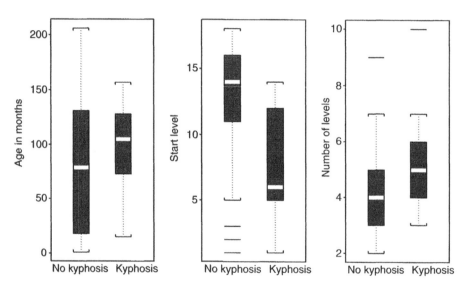

Figure 4.7   Boxplots for the three risk factors in the kyphosis data.

the vertical, following surgery – age in months, the starting vertebral level of the surgery (start) and the number of vertebrae involved (number) – and the objective was to determine which of these are important. Hastie and Tibshirani (1990) give a very detailed analysis of these data. Here we shall content ourselves with examining relatively briefly how a number of GAMs can be applied to the observations.

It is useful to begin the exploration of the kyphosis data with boxplots for the two levels of the response variable for each of the three risk factors. These are shown in Figure 4.7. The plots show a location shift for all three risk factors, and a number of possible outliers in the plots involving start level and number of levels. We shall, however, retain all the observations in the subsequent analyses.

We next fit a GAM using a logistic link function for the expected value of the response variable, and cubic spline terms for each of the three explanatory variables.

Table 4.7 Results of fitting a GAM model with cubic splines and logistic regression to kyphosis data

(a) GAM

	df npar.	*df npar.*	χ^2	$Pr(\chi^2)$
s(Age)	1	2.9	5.783	0.116
s(Start)	1	2.9	5.806	0.114
s(Number)	1	3.0	5.656	0.130

(b) Logistic regression

Covariate	*Estimated regression coefficient*	*Standard error*	*Estimate/SE*
Age	0.011	0.006	1.696
Start	−0.207	0.068	−3.051
Number	0.411	0.225	1.827

(c) Comparison of models

Terms	*Resid. df*	*Resid. dev*	*Test*	*df*	*Deviance*
Age + Start + Number	77.00000	61.37993			
s(Age) + s(Start) + s(Number)	68.19092	40.75528	1 vs. 2	8.80901	20.62465

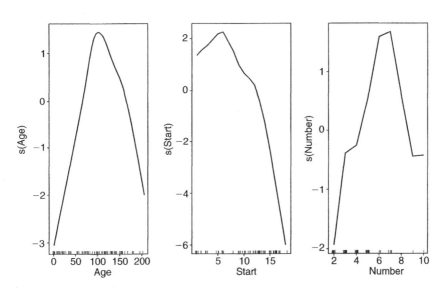

Figure 4.8 Cubic spline functions for each risk factor in the kyphosis data.

The results are shown in Table 4.7. The evidence for nonlinearity in any of the variables is not strong. A plot of the fitted functions is shown in Figure 4.8.

Also given in Table 4.7 is a comparison of the GAM fit with the fit of a logistic regression model which includes simple linear effects for each of the three explanatory variables. Judging the decrease in deviance as a chi-square with 9 df, the associated *p*-value is 0.014, indicating that the model allowing for nonlinear effects fits the data best. Investigating whether nonlinear terms are needed for all the three risk factors is left as an exercise for the reader (see Exercise 4.2).

4.5   Summary

Generalized additive models provide a useful addition to the tools available for exploring the relationship between a response variable and a set of explanatory variables. Such models allow possible nonlinear terms in the latter to be uncovered, and perhaps then to be modelled in terms of more familiar low-degree polynomials. The GAM model can deal with nonlinearity in covariates that are not the main interest in a study, and 'adjust' for those effects appropriately.

Software

Software for fitting GAMs is not as widely available as that for GLMs but is gradually becoming easier to find. Some examples of what is available are the following:

SAS   proc gam (experimental in version 8.1, 'production' in version 8.2);
S-PLUS   The gam function

(Details on the fitting of GAM models using S-PLUS are given in Everitt, 2001.)

Table 4.8   Erythrocyte sedimentation rate data for Exercise 4.4

Fibrinogen	Gamma	ESR	Fibrinogen	Gamma	ESR
2.52	38	0	3.53	46	1
2.56	31	0	2.68	34	0
2.19	33	0	2.60	38	0
2.18	31	0	2.23	37	0
3.41	37	0	2.88	30	0
2.46	36	0	2.65	46	0
3.22	38	0	2.09	44	1
2.21	37	0	2.28	36	0
3.15	39	0	2.67	39	0
2.60	41	0	2.29	31	0
2.29	36	0	2.15	31	0
2.35	29	0	2.54	28	0
5.06	37	1	3.93	32	1
3.34	32	1	3.34	30	0
2.38	37	1	2.99	36	0
3.15	36	0	3.32	35	0

Source: Collett and Jemain (1985).

Exercises

4.1 Fit a model to the insulin dependence data that allows a quadratic effect of age and a linear effect of base. Compare its fit with the GAMs fitted in the text.

4.2 Investigate whether nonlinear effects are necessary for all the risk factors in the kyphosis data.

4.3 Investigate the use of the GAMs on the hypertension data in Chapter 1 (Table 1.1).

4.4 The data in Table 4.8 are given in Collett and Jemain (1985), and concern the erythrocyte sedimentation rate (ESR), that is, the rate at which red blood cells (erythrocytes) settle out of suspension in blood plasma when measured under standard conditions. The ESR for a 'healthy' individual should be less than 20 mm/h, and the response variable in the data denotes whether this is the case (0 = less than 20, 1 = greater than 20). Assess how the probability of an ESR reading greater than 20 depends on the levels of the two proteins using (i) logistic regression and (ii) GAMs.

5

Classification and Regression Trees

5.1 Introduction

Previous chapters have dealt with a number of regression-type models, generalized linear models, mixed effects models and generalized additive models. Such methods are widely used, but they may not always give faithful data descriptions when the assumptions on which they are based are not met, or in the presence of higher-order interactions among some of the explanatory variables.

An entirely different approach to explaining the relationship between a response variable and a set of explanatory variables which has been developed to overcome some of these possible problems is the *classification and regression tree* (CART) procedure. The central theme of this approach is the extraction of subgroups of observations within which the explanatory variables are relatively homogeneous, and between which the response variable is relatively distinct. Creation of subgroups takes place according to a tree structure, in essence a series of *binary splits*. Often the resulting tree is readily interpretable and offers insight into the structure and pattern in the data.

Such tree structures have a long and relatively respectable history, with early examples being described in Morgan and Sonquist (1963) and Morgan and Messenger

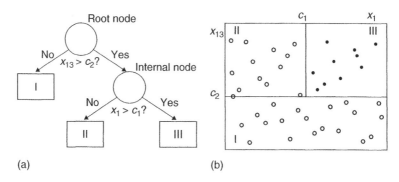

Figure 5.1 An illustrative tree structure. Circles and dots are different outcomes. (Taken from Zhang and Singer, 1999, with permission of the publisher, Springer-Verlag.)

(1973). Current tree methodology and software are largely based on original work by Breiman *et al.* (1984).

The basic ideas behind tree models are illustrated in Figure 5.1, taken from Zhang and Singer (1999). Here the tree is formed by two variables, and the tree has three layers of nodes. The first layer is the unique root mode, namely the circle at the top. One internal node (the other circle) is in the second layer, and the three terminal nodes (the boxes) are in the second and third layers. Both the root node and the internal node are partitioned into two nodes in the next layer, called *left* and *right daughter nodes*. By definition, however, the terminal nodes do not have offspring nodes. How parent nodes are split into two daughter nodes and when a terminal node is declared are questions that will be taken up in the next section.

5.2   Tree-based models

The underlying idea of tree techniques is the formation of subgroups of individuals within which the response variable is relatively homogeneous. Developing a tree model involves the construction of a collection of rules that eventually lead to the terminal nodes. An example of a rule for data consisting of a response variable y and a set of explanatory variables, $x_1 \ldots, x_p$ might be if $(x_2 < 410)$ and $(x_4 \in \{C,D,E\})$ and $(x_5 > 10)$ then the predicted value of y is 4.75 (if y is continuous), or, the probability that $y = 1$ is 0.7 (if y is binary).

The complete collection of rules that defines the tree is arrived at by a process known as *recursive partitioning*. A series of binary splits is made based on the answers to questions of the type 'Does observation or case $i \in A$?', where A is a region of the covariate space. Answering such a question induces a partition, or split, of the covariate space. Cases for which the answer is yes are assigned to one group, and those for which the answer is no to an alternative group.

Most implementations of tree modelling proceed by imposing the following constraints:

- Each split depends on the value of only a single covariate.
- For ordered (continuous or categorical) covariates x_j, only splits resulting from the questions of the form 'Is $x_j < C$?' are considered. Thus, ordering is preserved.
- For categorical explanatory variables, all possible splits into disjoint subsets of the categories are allowed.

A tree is grown as follows:

1. Examine every allowable split on each explanatory variable.
2. Select and execute (that is, create left and right daughter nodes) from the best of these splits.

The initial or root node of the tree comprises the whole sample. Steps 1 and 2 are then reapplied to each of the daughter nodes. Various procedures are used to control tree size, as we shall describe later.

To determine the best node to split into left and right daughter nodes at any stage in the construction of the tree involves the use of a numerical *split function*, $\phi(s, g)$, often referred to simply as deviance. This can be evaluated for any split s of node g. The form of $\phi(s, g)$ depends on whether the response variable is continuous or categorical.

The usual split function chosen for a continuous response variable is based on the *within-node sum of squares*, that is for a node g with N_g cases, the term

$$SS(g) = \sum_{i \in g} [y_i - \bar{y}(g)]^2 \tag{5.1}$$

where y_i denotes the response variable value for the ith individual and $\bar{y}(g)$ is the mean of the responses of the N_g cases in node g. If a particular split, s, of node g is into left and right daughter nodes, g_L and g_R, then the least-squares split function is given by

$$\phi(s, g) = SS(g) - SS(g_L) - SS(g_R) \tag{5.2}$$

and the best split of node g is determined as the one that corresponds to the maximum of (5.2) amongst all allowable splits.

Split functions for categorical response variables (in particular, binary variables) are based on trying to make the probability of a particular category of the variable close to one or zero in each node. Most commonly used is a log-likelihood function defined for node g as

$$LL(g) = -2 \sum_{i \in g} \sum_{k=1}^{K} y_{ik} \log(p_{gk}) \tag{5.3}$$

where K is the number of categories of the response variable, y_{ik} is an indicator variable taking the value 1 if individual i is in category k of the response and zero otherwise, and p_{gk} is the probability of being in the kth category of the response in node g, estimated as n_{gk}/N_g, where n_{gk} is the number of individuals in category k in node g. The corresponding split function $\phi(s, g)$ is then calculated as

$$\phi(s, g) = LL(g) - LL(g_L) - LL(g_k) \tag{5.4}$$

and again the chosen split is that maximizing $\phi(s, g)$.

Trees are grown by recursively splitting nodes to maximize ϕ, leading to smaller and smaller nodes of progressively increased homogeneity. A critical question is when tree construction should end and terminal nodes be declared. Two simple 'stopping' rules are:

- *Node size* – stop when this drops below a threshold value, for example, when $N_g < 10$.
- *Node homogeneity* – stop when a node is homogeneous enough, for example, when its deviance is less than 1% of the deviance of the root node.

Neither of these is particularly attractive because they have to be judged relative to preset thresholds, misspecification of which can result in overfitting or underfitting. An alternative, more complex approach is to use what is known as a *pruning algorithm*. This involves growing a very large initial tree to capture all potentially important splits, and then collapsing this back up using what is known as *cost complexity pruning* to create a nested sequence of trees.

Cost complexity pruning is a procedure which snips off the least important splits in the initial tree, where importance is judged by a measure of within-node homogeneity or *cost*. For a continuous variable, for example, cost would simply be the sum-of-squares term defined in (5.1). The cost of the entire tree, G, is then defined as

$$\text{Cost}(G) = \sum_{g \in G} SS(g) \tag{5.5}$$

where $\widetilde{G}$ is the collection of terminal nodes of G. Next we define the complexity of G as the number of its terminal nodes, say $N_{\widetilde{G}}$ and finally, we can define the *cost complexity* of G as

$$CC_\alpha(G) = \text{Cost}(G) + \alpha N_{\widetilde{G}} \qquad (5.6)$$

where $\alpha \geq 0$ is called the *complexity parameter*. The aim is to minimize simultaneously both cost and complexity; large trees will have small cost but high complexity, with the reverse being the case for small trees. Solely minimizing cost will err on the side of overfitting; for example, with $SS(g)$ we can achieve zero cost by splitting to a point where each terminal node contains only a single observation. In practice, we use (5.6) by considering a range of values of α and for each find the subtree $G(\alpha)$ of our initial tree that minimizes $CC_\alpha(G)$. If α is small $G(\alpha)$ will be large, and as α increases, $N_{\widetilde{G}}$ decreases. For a sufficiently large α, $N_{\widetilde{G}} = 1$.

In this way we are led to a sequence of possible trees and need to consider how to select the best. There are two possibilities:

- If a separate validation sample is available, we can predict on that set of observations and calculate the deviance versus α for the pruned trees. This will often have a minimum, and so the smallest tree whose sum of squares is close to the minimum can be chosen.
- If no validation set is available, one can be constructed from the observations used in constructing the tree, by splitting the observations into a number of subsets of (roughly) equal size. If n subsets are formed this way, $n - 1$ can be used to grow the tree and it can be tested on the remaining subset. This can be done n ways, and the results averaged.

Now let us move on to consider applications of tree-based models in a particular area, namely, the birthweight of babies.

5.3 Birthweight of babies

The birthweight of babies is often a useful indicator of how they will thrive in the first few months of their life. Low birthweight, say below 2.5 kg, is often a cause of concern for their welfare. Hosmer and Lemeshow (1989) describe a data set collected to investigate which of a number of factors may be predictive of birthweight. The data are given in Table 5.1 and show the following for each of 189 births in a hospital in the USA:

low	–	a binary variable indicating whether birthweight was below 2.5 kg
age	–	age of mother in years
lwt	–	weight of mother (lbs) at last menstrual period
race	–	white, black or other
smoke	–	a binary variable indicating smoking status during pregnancy
ptl	–	number of previous premature labours
ht	–	a binary variable indicating history of hypertension
ui	–	a binary variable indicating whether mother has uterine irritability
ftv	–	number of physician visits in the first trimester
bwt	–	actual birthweight (grams)

To begin, suppose we consider *low* as a binary response variable. Before applying a tree model, we might examine the results of a more usual method of analysis for

Table 5.1   Birthweight of babies

Baby	low	age	lwt	race	smoke	ptl	ht	ui	ftv	bwt
1	ge2.5	19	182	black	ns	0	nht	ui	0	2523
2	ge2.5	33	155	other	ns	0	nht	nui	3	2551
3	ge2.5	20	105	white	s	0	nht	nui	1	2557
4	ge2.5	21	108	white	s	0	nht	ui	2	2594
5	ge2.5	18	107	white	s	0	nht	ui	0	2600
6	ge2.5	21	124	other	ns	0	nht	nui	0	2622
7	ge2.5	22	118	white	ns	0	nht	nui	1	2637
8	ge2.5	17	103	other	ns	0	nht	nui	1	2637
9	ge2.5	29	123	white	s	0	nht	nui	1	2663
10	ge2.5	26	113	white	s	0	nht	nui	0	2665
11	ge2.5	19	95	other	ns	0	nht	nui	0	2722
12	ge2.5	19	150	other	ns	0	nht	nui	1	2733
13	ge2.5	22	95	other	ns	0	ht	nui	0	2751
14	ge2.5	30	107	other	ns	1	nht	ui	2	2750
15	ge2.5	18	100	white	s	0	nht	nui	0	2769
16	ge2.5	18	100	white	s	0	nht	nui	0	2769
17	ge2.5	15	98	black	ns	0	nht	nui	0	2778
18	ge2.5	25	118	white	s	0	nht	nui	3	2782
19	ge2.5	20	120	other	ns	0	nht	ui	0	2807
20	ge2.5	28	120	white	s	0	nht	nui	1	2821
21	ge2.5	32	121	other	ns	0	nht	nui	2	2835
22	ge2.5	31	100	white	ns	0	nht	ui	3	2835
23	ge2.5	36	202	white	ns	0	nht	nui	1	2836
24	ge2.5	28	120	other	ns	0	nht	nui	0	2863
25	ge2.5	25	120	other	ns	0	nht	ui	2	2877
26	ge2.5	28	167	white	ns	0	nht	nui	0	2877
27	ge2.5	17	122	white	s	0	nht	nui	0	2906
28	ge2.5	29	150	white	ns	0	nht	nui	2	2920
29	ge2.5	26	168	black	s	0	nht	nui	0	2920
30	ge2.5	17	113	black	ns	0	nht	nui	1	2920
31	ge2.5	17	113	black	ns	0	nht	nui	1	2920
32	ge2.5	24	90	white	s	1	nht	nui	1	2948
33	ge2.5	35	121	black	s	1	nht	nui	1	2948
34	ge2.5	25	155	white	ns	0	nht	nui	1	2977
35	ge2.5	25	125	black	ns	0	nht	nui	0	2977
36	ge2.5	29	140	white	s	0	nht	nui	2	2977
37	ge2.5	19	138	white	s	0	nht	nui	2	2977
38	ge2.5	27	124	white	s	0	nht	nui	0	2922
39	ge2.5	31	215	white	s	0	nht	nui	2	3005
40	ge2.5	33	109	white	s	0	nht	nui	1	3033
41	ge2.5	21	185	black	s	0	nht	nui	2	3042
42	ge2.5	19	189	white	ns	0	nht	nui	2	3062
43	ge2.5	23	130	black	ns	0	nht	nui	1	3062
44	ge2.5	21	160	white	ns	0	nht	nui	0	3062
45	ge2.5	18	90	white	s	0	nht	ui	0	3062
46	ge2.5	18	90	white	s	0	nht	ui	0	3062
47	ge2.5	32	132	white	ns	0	nht	nui	4	3080
48	ge2.5	19	132	other	ns	0	nht	nui	0	3090
49	ge2.5	24	115	white	ns	0	nht	nui	2	3090
50	ge2.5	22	85	other	s	0	nht	nui	0	3090
51	ge2.5	22	120	white	ns	0	ht	nui	1	3100
52	ge2.5	23	128	other	ns	0	nht	nui	0	3104
53	ge2.5	22	130	white	s	0	nht	nui	0	3132

(*Continued*)

Table 5.1 (*Continued*)

Baby	low	age	lwt	race	smoke	ptl	ht	ui	ftv	bwt
54	ge2.5	30	95	white	s	0	nht	nui	2	3147
55	ge2.5	19	115	other	ns	0	nht	nui	0	3175
56	ge2.5	16	110	other	ns	0	nht	nui	0	3175
57	ge2.5	21	110	other	s	0	nht	ui	0	3203
58	ge2.5	30	153	other	ns	0	nht	nui	0	3203
59	ge2.5	20	103	other	ns	0	nht	nui	0	3203
60	ge2.5	17	119	other	ns	0	nht	nui	0	3225
61	ge2.5	17	119	other	ns	0	nht	nui	0	3225
62	ge2.5	23	119	other	ns	0	nht	nui	2	3232
63	ge2.5	24	110	other	ns	0	nht	nui	0	3232
64	ge2.5	28	140	white	ns	0	nht	nui	0	3234
65	ge2.5	26	133	other	s	2	nht	nui	0	3260
66	ge2.5	20	169	other	ns	1	nht	ui	1	3274
67	ge2.5	24	115	other	ns	0	nht	nui	2	3274
68	ge2.5	28	250	other	s	0	nht	nui	6	3303
69	ge2.5	20	141	white	ns	2	nht	ui	1	3317
70	ge2.5	22	158	black	ns	1	nht	nui	2	3317
71	ge2.5	22	112	white	s	2	nht	nui	0	3317
72	ge2.5	31	150	other	s	0	nht	nui	2	3321
73	ge2.5	23	115	other	s	0	nht	nui	1	3331
74	ge2.5	16	112	black	ns	0	nht	nui	0	3374
75	ge2.5	16	135	white	s	0	nht	nui	0	3374
76	ge2.5	18	229	black	ns	0	nht	nui	0	3402
77	ge2.5	25	140	white	ns	0	nht	nui	1	3416
78	ge2.5	32	134	white	s	1	nht	nui	4	3430
79	ge2.5	20	121	black	s	0	nht	nui	0	3444
80	ge2.5	23	190	white	ns	0	nht	nui	0	3459
81	ge2.5	22	131	white	ns	0	nht	nui	1	3460
82	ge2.5	32	170	white	ns	0	nht	nui	0	3473
83	ge2.5	30	110	other	ns	0	nht	nui	0	3544
84	ge2.5	20	127	other	ns	0	nht	nui	0	3487
85	ge2.5	23	123	other	ns	0	nht	nui	0	3544
86	ge2.5	17	120	other	s	0	nht	nui	0	3572
87	ge2.5	19	105	other	ns	0	nht	nui	0	3572
88	ge2.5	23	130	white	ns	0	nht	nui	0	3586
89	ge2.5	36	175	white	ns	0	nht	nui	0	3600
90	ge2.5	22	125	white	ns	0	nht	nui	1	3614
91	ge2.5	24	133	white	ns	0	nht	nui	0	3614
92	ge2.5	21	134	other	ns	0	nht	nui	2	3629
93	ge2.5	19	235	white	s	0	ht	nui	0	3629
94	ge2.5	25	95	white	s	3	nht	ui	0	3637
95	ge2.5	16	135	white	s	0	nht	nui	0	3643
96	ge2.5	29	135	white	ns	0	nht	nui	1	3651
97	ge2.5	29	154	white	ns	0	nht	nui	1	3651
98	ge2.5	19	147	white	s	0	nht	nui	0	3651
99	ge2.5	19	147	white	s	0	nht	nui	0	3651
100	ge2.5	30	137	white	ns	0	nht	nui	1	3699
101	ge2.5	24	110	white	ns	0	nht	nui	1	3728
102	ge2.5	19	184	white	s	0	ht	nui	0	3756
103	ge2.5	24	110	other	ns	1	nht	nui	0	3770
104	ge2.5	23	110	white	ns	0	nht	nui	1	3770
105	ge2.5	20	120	other	ns	0	nht	nui	0	3770

(*Continued*)

Table 5.1 (*Continued*)

Baby	low	age	lwt	race	smoke	ptl	ht	ui	ftv	bwt
106	ge2.5	25	241	black	ns	0	ht	nui	0	3790
107	ge2.5	30	112	white	ns	0	nht	nui	1	3799
108	ge2.5	22	169	white	ns	0	nht	nui	0	3827
109	ge2.5	18	120	white	s	0	nht	nui	2	3856
110	ge2.5	16	170	black	ns	0	nht	nui	4	3860
111	ge2.5	32	186	white	ns	0	nht	nui	2	3860
112	ge2.5	18	120	other	ns	0	nht	nui	1	3884
113	ge2.5	29	130	white	s	0	nht	nui	2	3884
114	ge2.5	33	117	white	ns	0	nht	ui	1	3912
115	ge2.5	20	170	white	s	0	nht	nui	0	3940
116	ge2.5	28	134	other	ns	0	nht	nui	1	3941
117	ge2.5	14	135	white	ns	0	nht	nui	0	3941
118	ge2.5	28	130	other	ns	0	nht	nui	0	3969
119	ge2.5	25	120	white	ns	0	nht	nui	2	3983
120	ge2.5	16	95	other	ns	0	nht	nui	1	3997
121	ge2.5	20	158	white	ns	0	nht	nui	1	3997
122	ge2.5	26	160	other	ns	0	nht	nui	0	4054
123	ge2.5	21	115	white	ns	0	nht	nui	1	4054
124	ge2.5	22	129	white	ns	0	nht	nui	0	4111
125	ge2.5	25	130	white	ns	0	nht	nui	2	4153
126	ge2.5	31	120	white	ns	0	nht	nui	2	4167
127	ge2.5	35	170	white	ns	1	nht	nui	1	4174
128	ge2.5	19	120	white	s	0	nht	nui	0	4238
129	ge2.5	24	116	white	ns	0	nht	nui	1	4593
130	ge2.5	45	123	white	ns	0	nht	nui	1	4990
131	le2.5	28	120	other	s	1	nht	ui	0	709
132	le2.5	29	130	white	ns	0	nht	ui	2	1021
133	le2.5	34	187	black	s	0	ht	nui	0	1135
134	le2.5	25	105	other	ns	1	ht	nui	0	1330
135	le2.5	25	85	other	ns	0	nht	ui	0	1474
136	le2.5	27	150	other	ns	0	nht	nui	0	1588
137	le2.5	23	97	other	ns	0	nht	ui	1	1588
138	le2.5	24	128	black	ns	1	nht	nui	1	1701
139	le2.5	24	132	other	ns	0	ht	nui	0	1729
140	le2.5	21	165	white	s	0	ht	nui	1	1790
141	le2.5	32	105	white	s	0	nht	nui	0	1818
142	le2.5	19	91	white	s	2	nht	ui	0	1885
143	le2.5	25	115	other	ns	0	nht	nui	0	1893
144	le2.5	16	130	other	ns	0	nht	nui	1	1899
145	le2.5	25	92	white	s	0	nht	nui	0	1928
146	le2.5	20	150	white	s	0	nht	nui	2	1928
147	le2.5	21	200	black	ns	0	nht	ui	2	1928
148	le2.5	24	155	white	s	1	nht	nui	0	1936
149	le2.5	21	103	other	ns	0	nht	nui	0	1970
150	le2.5	20	125	other	ns	0	nht	ui	0	2055
151	le2.5	25	89	other	ns	2	nht	nui	1	2055
152	le2.5	19	102	white	ns	0	nht	nui	2	2082
153	le2.5	19	112	white	s	0	nht	ui	0	2084
154	le2.5	26	117	white	s	1	nht	nui	0	2084
155	le2.5	24	138	white	ns	0	nht	nui	0	2100
156	le2.5	17	130	other	s	1	nht	ui	0	2125
157	le2.5	20	120	black	s	0	nht	nui	3	2126

(*Continued*)

Table 5.1 (*Continued*)

Baby	low	age	lwt	race	smoke	ptl	ht	ui	ftv	bwt
158	1e2.5	22	130	white	s	1	nht	ui	1	2187
159	1e2.5	27	130	black	ns	0	nht	ui	0	2187
160	1e2.5	20	80	other	s	0	nht	ui	0	2211
161	1e2.5	17	110	white	s	0	nht	nui	0	2225
162	1e2.5	25	105	other	ns	1	nht	nui	1	2240
163	1e2.5	20	109	other	ns	0	nht	nui	0	2240
164	1e2.5	18	148	other	ns	0	nht	nui	0	2282
165	1e2.5	18	110	black	s	1	nht	nui	0	2296
166	1e2.5	20	121	white	s	1	nht	ui	0	2296
167	1e2.5	21	100	other	ns	1	nht	nui	4	2301
168	1e2.5	26	96	other	ns	0	nht	nui	0	2325
169	1e2.5	31	102	white	s	1	nht	nui	1	2353
170	1e2.5	15	110	white	ns	0	nht	nui	0	2353
171	1e2.5	23	187	black	s	0	nht	nui	1	2367
172	1e2.5	20	122	black	s	0	nht	nui	0	2381
173	1e2.5	24	105	black	s	0	nht	nui	0	2381
174	1e2.5	15	115	other	ns	0	nht	ui	0	2381
175	1e2.5	23	120	other	ns	0	nht	nui	0	2410
176	1e2.5	30	142	white	s	1	nht	nui	0	2410
177	1e2.5	22	130	white	s	0	nht	nui	1	2410
178	1e2.5	17	120	white	s	0	nht	nui	3	2414
179	1e2.5	23	110	white	s	1	nht	nui	0	2424
180	1e2.5	17	120	black	ns	0	nht	nui	2	2438
181	1e2.5	26	154	other	ns	1	ht	nui	1	2442
182	1e2.5	20	105	other	ns	0	nht	nui	3	2450
183	1e2.5	26	190	white	s	0	nht	nui	0	2466
184	1e2.5	14	101	other	s	1	nht	nui	0	2466
185	1e2.5	28	95	white	s	0	nht	nui	2	2466
186	1e2.5	14	100	other	ns	0	nht	nui	2	2495
187	1e2.5	23	94	other	s	0	nht	nui	0	2495
188	1e2.5	17	142	black	ns	0	ht	nui	0	2495
189	1e2.5	21	130	white	s	0	ht	nui	3	2495

such a variable, namely logistic regression. The results of fitting such a model to *low* using all but actual birthweight as covariates are shown in Table 5.2. (Race has been coded in terms of two dummy variables in this analysis.) Mother's weight, race, smoking status and history of hypertension all appear to be potentially useful predictors of whether birthweight is below 2.5 kg, although a detailed analysis would be required to identify which of these covariates were most predictive – we leave this as an exercise for the reader (see Exercise 5.1).

Now let us move on to apply tree models to these data; since the response here is categorical, the associated trees are generally known as *classification trees*. We begin with some very simple models involving only one or two of the explanatory variables, so that the concepts behind the construction of trees can be clarified. Using only smoking status, for example, results in the tree described in Table 5.3. The root node contains all 189 subjects; it is from this node that the tree is grown. Thereafter, nodes of the tree contain subsets of the root node sample. Here the only possible division is into smokers ($n = 74$) and non-smokers ($n = 115$). For the latter, the probability of

Table 5.2   Results of fitting a logistic regression model to the binary variable *low*

Covariate	Estimated regression coefficient	Standard error	Estimate/SE
Intercept	2.983	1.247	2.392
Age	−0.030	0.037	−0.798
lwt	−0.015	0.007	−2.230
Race 1	0.636	0.264	2.413
Race 2	0.081	0.138	0.589
Smoke	0.469	0.201	2.335
plt	0.543	0.345	1.573
ht	0.932	0.3489	2.672
ui	0.384	0.230	1.672
ftv	0.065	0.172	0.379

(Dispersion parameter for binomial family taken to be 1.)
Null deviance: 234.67 on 188 degrees of freedom.
Residual deviance: 201.28 on 179 degrees of freedom.

Table 5.3   Classification tree for *low* using only smoking status as an explanatory variable

node), split, n, deviance, yval, (yprob)
1) root 189 234.670 ge2.5 (0.68783 0.31217)
  2) smoke:ns 115 129.880 ge2.5 (0.74783 0.25217)*
  3) smoke:s 74 99.921 ge2.5 (0.59459 0.40541)*

* denotes terminal node.

giving birth to a baby above 2.5 kg in weight is estimated to be 0.75, for the former 0.59. The deviance of the root node, 234.67, arises from calculating

$$-2[130\log(130/189) + 59\log(59/189)] \tag{5.7}$$

Similarly, the deviance value for smokers, 99.92, is the result of calculating

$$-2[44\log(44/74) + 30\log(30/74)] \tag{5.8}$$

and that for non-smokers, 129.88, is derived from

$$-2[86\log(86/115) + 29\log(29/115)] \tag{5.9}$$

Now consider the classification tree for the continuous variable, *age*. Age has 23 distinct values in the range 14 to 36. Hence it leads to $23 - 1 = 22$ allowable splits. One split, for example, can be whether age is more than 20 years. In general, for an ordinal or a continuous explanatory variable, the number of allowable splits is one fewer than the number of its distinctly observed values. The classification tree for the response variable *low*, using the single explanatory variable *age*, is shown in Table 5.4, and in graphical form in Figure 5.2. Things have now become a little more complicated! The first split is into mothers less than 28 years of age (146) and those 28 and older (43). The left-hand daughter node is then split at 16, and the right-hand daughter node

Table 5.4   Classification tree for response variable *low* using age as an explanatory variable

```
node), split, n, deviance, yval, (yprob)

 1) root 189 234.6700 ge2.5 ( 0.68783 0.31217 )
   2) age<27.5 146 190.1400 ge2.5 ( 0.64384 0.35616 )
     4) age<15.5 6    7.6382 le2.5 ( 0.33333 0.66667 ) *
     5) age>15.5 140 180.0200 ge2.5 ( 0.65714 0.34286 )
      10) age<19.5 45   50.0530 ge2.5 ( 0.75556 0.24444 )
        20) age<17.5 19   23.6990 ge2.5 ( 0.68421 0.31579 )
          40) age<16.5 7    5.7416 ge2.5 ( 0.85714 0.14286 ) *
          41) age>16.5 12   16.3010 ge2.5 ( 0.58333 0.41667 ) *
        21) age>17.5 26   25.4570 ge2.5 ( 0.80769 0.19231 )
          42) age<18.5 10   10.0080 ge2.5 ( 0.80000 0.20000 ) *
          43) age>18.5 16   15.4420 ge2.5 ( 0.81250 0.18750 ) *
      11) age>19.5 95 127.0200 ge2.5 ( 0.61053 0.38947 )
        22) age<25.5 84 110.6200 ge2.5 ( 0.63095 0.36905 )
          44) age<21.5 30   41.0540 ge2.5 ( 0.56667 0.43333 )
            88) age<20.5 18   24.7310 ge2.5 ( 0.55556 0.44444 ) *
            89) age>20.5 12   16.3010 ge2.5 ( 0.58333 0.41667 ) *
          45) age>21.5 54   68.7440 ge2.5 ( 0.66667 0.33333 )
            90) age<22.5 13   11.1620 ge2.5 ( 0.84615 0.15385 ) *
            91) age>22.5 41   54.8460 ge2.5 ( 0.60976 0.39024 )
             182) age<24.5 26   34.6460 ge2.5 ( 0.61538 0.38462 )
               364) age<23.5 13   17.3230 ge2.5 ( 0.61538 0.38462 ) *
               365) age>23.5 13   17.3230 ge2.5 ( 0.61538 0.38462 ) *
             183) age>24.5 15   20.1900 ge2.5 ( 0.60000 0.40000 ) *
        23) age>25.5 11   15.1580 le2.5 ( 0.45455 0.54545 ) *
   3) age>27.5 43   38.2070 ge2.5 ( 0.83721 0.16279 )
     6) age<34.5 38   36.3070 ge2.5 ( 0.81579 0.18421 )
      12) age<28.5 9    9.5347 ge2.5 ( 0.77778 0.22222 ) *
      13) age>28.5 29   26.6620 ge2.5 ( 0.82759 0.17241 )
        26) age<30.5 14   11.4830 ge2.5 ( 0.85714 0.14286 )
          52) age<29.5 7    5.7416 ge2.5 ( 0.85714 0.14286 ) *
          53) age>29.5 7    5.7416 ge2.5 ( 0.85714 0.14286 ) *
        27) age>30.5 15   15.0120 ge2.5 ( 0.80000 0.20000 )
          54) age<31.5 5    5.0040 ge2.5 ( 0.80000 0.20000 ) *
          55) age>31.5 10   10.0080 ge2.5 ( 0.80000 0.20000 ) *
     7) age>34.5 5    0.0000 ge2.5 ( 1.00000 0.00000 ) *
```

*denotes terminal node.

at 35. Terminal nodes are indicated by rectangles, and nodes are labelled by the majority category of the two categories of *low*. The properties given below each node indicate the value for the minority category in the node.

Now let us consider actual birthweight as the response variable. First, the results of fitting a multiple regression model for this response using all the other variables except for *low* as covariates are shown in Table 5.5. Again race, smoking status, mother's weight and history of hypertension appear to be potential predictors.

Using *smoke* as a single explanatory variable to construct our first *regression tree* for birthweight gives the results shown in Table 5.6. The average birthweight for babies of smokers is 2771.9 g and for non-smokers 3055.7 g. In this case the deviance is simply the corrected sum of squares for the birthweights of the individuals in a node, that is, the within-node sum of squares for birthweight.

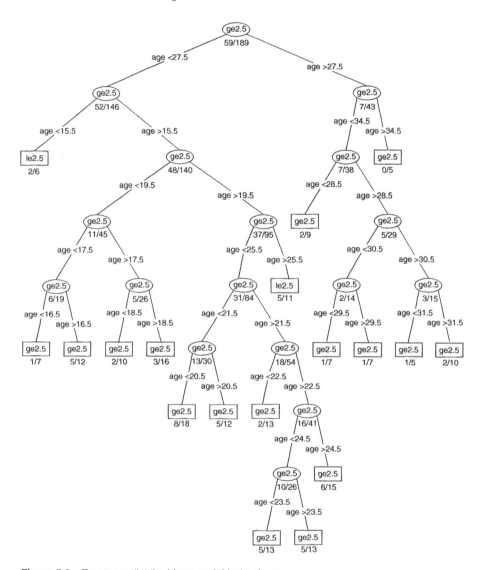

Figure 5.2   Tree to predict the binary variable *low* from age.

A slightly more interesting tree results from using *race* with three unordered categories. Here, the allowable splits from the root node are {white: black and other}, {black:
white and other}, and {other: white and black}. These three splits are considered, and
the one that maximizes ϕ, as defined earlier, is selected. This leads to the tree shown
in Table 5.7. A graphic representation of the tree helps here – see Figure 5.3. From
the root node, the first split is {white: black, other}, and then a further split of the
black/other node is made. Here, the regression tree simply orders average birthweights:
black 2719.7 g, other 2805.3 g, white 3102.7 g.

Now, let us examine the regression-tree approach for birthweight and two explanatory variables, *smoke* and *race*. Details of the tree are given in Table 5.8, and the tree

Table 5.5 Results of fitting a multiple regression model to actual birthweight

Covariate	Estimated regression coefficient	Standard error	Estimate/SE
Intercept	1916.317	313.904	6.105
Age	−3.570	9.620	−0.371
lwt	4.354	1.736	2.509
Race 1	−244.214	74.992	−3.257
Race 2	−36.954	38.964	−0.948
Smoke	−176.022	53.238	−3.306
plt	−48.402	101.972	−0.475
ht	−296.414	101.161	−2.930
ui	−258.040	69.443	−3.716
ftv	−14.058	46.468	−0.303

Residual standard error: 650.3 on 179 degrees of freedom.
Multiple R-squared: 0.243.
F-statistic: 6.376 on 9 and 179 degrees of freedom, the p-value is <0.0001.

Table 5.6 Regression tree for birthweight with smoke as a single explanatory variable

node), split, n, deviance, yval

1) root 189 99970000 2944.6
   2) smoke:s 74 31764000 2771.9*
   3) smoke:ns 115 64580000 3055.7*

* denotes terminal node.

Table 5.7 Regression tree for birthweight using race as a single explanatory variable

node), split, n, deviance, yval

1) root 189 99970000 2944.6
   2) race:black,other 93 44758000 2781.4
     4) race:black 26 10198000 2719.7*
     5) race:other 67 34423000 2805.3*
   3) race:white 96 50333000 3102.7*

* denotes terminal node.

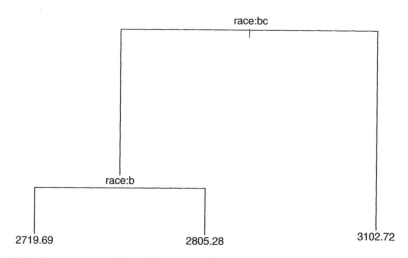

race:bc

race:b

2719.69   2805.28   3102.72

Figure 5.3 Tree to predict birthweight from ethnicity.

Table 5.8 Regression tree for birthweight using race and smoking status as explanatory variables

```
node), split, n, deviance, yval

1) root 189 99970000 2944.6
  2) race:black,other 93 44758000 2781.4
    4) smoke:s 22 11220000 2642.1
      8) race:black 10  3652600 2504.0 *
      9) race:other 12  7217900 2757.2 *
    5) smoke:ns 71 32979000 2824.5
      10) race:other 55 27172000 2815.8 *
      11) race:black 16  5789400 2854.5 *
  3) race:white 96 50333000 3102.7
    6) smoke:s 52 20016000 2826.8 *
    7) smoke:ns 44 21682000 3428.8 *
```

*denotes terminal node.

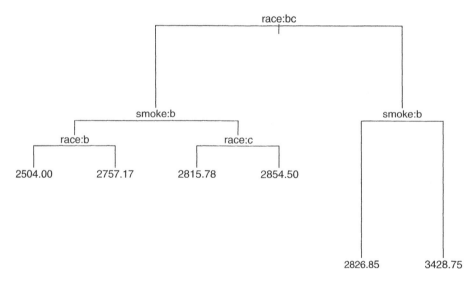

Figure 5.4 Tree to predict birthweight from ethnicity and smoking.

is displayed graphically in Figure 5.4. Here, the first split is on race into white and black/other. Each of the new nodes is then further split on the smoke variable into smokers and non-smokers, and then, on the left-hand side of the tree, further nodes are introduced by splitting race into black and other. The six terminal nodes and their average birthweights are as follows:

1. black, smokers: 2504, $n = 10$;
2. other, smokers: 2757, $n = 12$;
3. other, non-smokers: 2816, $n = 55$;
4. black, non-smokers: 2854, $n = 16$;

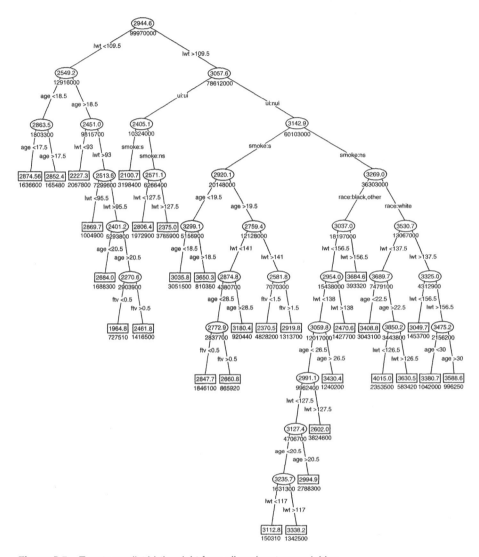

Figure 5.5 Tree to predict birthweight from all explanatory variables.

5. white, smokers: 2827, $n = 52$;
6. white, non-smokers: 3429, $n = 44$.

There is evidence here of a race × smoke interaction, at least for black and other women. Among smokers, black women produce babies with lower average birthweight than do 'other' women. But for non-smokers the reverse is the case.

Using all explanatory variables, the initial regression tree for birthweight is as shown in Table 5.9. The tree is graphed in Figure 5.5. The tree is complex, and we shall try to find a simplified version using the cost complexity pruning algorithm and cross-validation on the original data using a 10-fold split. The deviance against size

Table 5.9 Regression tree for birthweight using all covariates

```
node), split, n, deviance, yval

  1) root 189 99970000 2944.6
    2) lwt<109.5 42 12916000 2549.2
      4) age<18.5 10  1803300 2863.5
        8) age<17.5 5  1636600 2874.6 *
        9) age>17.5 5   165480 2852.4 *
      5) age>18.5 32  9815700 2451.0
       10) lwt<93 7  2067800 2227.3 *
       11) lwt>93 25  7299600 2513.6
         22) lwt<95.5 6  1004900 2869.7 *
         23) lwt>95.5 19  5293800 2401.2
           46) age<20.5 6  1688300 2684.0 *
           47) age>20.5 13  2903900 2270.6
             94) ftv<0.5 5   727510 1964.8 *
             95) ftv>0.5 8  1416500 2461.8 *
    3) lwt>109.5 147 78612000 3057.6
      6) ui:ui 17 10324000 2405.1
       12) smoke:s 6  3198400 2100.7 *
       13) smoke:ns 11  6266400 2571.1
         26) lwt<127.5 5  1972900 2806.4 *
         27) lwt>127.5 6  3785900 2375.0 *
      7) ui:nui 130 60103000 3142.9
       14) smoke:s 47 20148000 2920.1
         28) age<19.5 14  5156900 3299.1
           56) age<18.5 8  3051500 3035.8 *
           57) age>18.5 6   810350 3650.3 *
         29) age>19.5 33 12128000 2759.4
           58) lwt<141 20  4380700 2874.8
            116) age<28.5 15  2837700 2772.9
              232) ftv<0.5 9  1846100 2847.7 *
              233) ftv>0.5 6   865920 2660.8 *
            117) age>28.5 5   920440 3180.4 *
           59) lwt>141 13  7070300 2581.8
            118) ftv<1.5 8  4828200 2370.5 *
            119) ftv>1.5 5  1313700 2919.8 *
       15) smoke:ns 83 36303000 3269.0
         30) race:black,other 44 18197000 3037.0
           60) lwt<156.5 39 15438000 2954.0
            120) lwt<138 32 12017000 3059.8
              240) age<26.5 27  9962400 2991.1
                480) lwt<127.5 20  4706700 3127.4
                  960) age<20.5 11  1631300 3235.7
                   1920) lwt<117 5   150310 3112.8 *
                   1921) lwt>117 6  1342500 3338.2 *
                  961) age>20.5 9  2788300 2994.9 *
                481) lwt>127.5 7  3824600 2602.0 *
              241) age>26.5 5  1240200 3430.4 *
            121) lwt>138 7  1427700 2470.6 *
           61) lwt>156.5 5   393320 3684.6 *
         31) race:white 39 13067000 3530.7
           62) lwt<137.5 22  7479100 3689.7
            124) age<22.5 8  3043100 3408.8 *
            125) age>22.5 14  3443800 3850.2
              250) lwt<126.5 8  2353500 4015.0 *
              251) lwt>126.5 6   583420 3630.5 *
           63) lwt>137.5 17  4312900 3325.0
            126) lwt<156.5 6  1453700 3049.7 *
            127) lwt>156.5 11  2156200 3475.2
              254) age<30 6  1042000 3380.7 *
              255) age>30 5   996250 3588.6 *
```

* denotes terminal node.

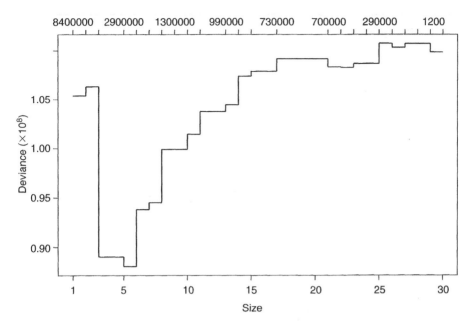

Figure 5.6   Deviance against size diagram for birthweight trees.

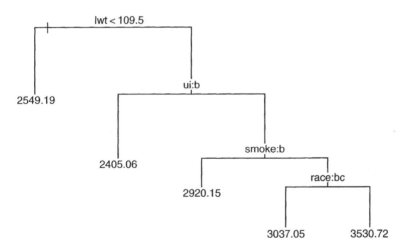

Figure 5.7   Optimal tree of size 5 for birthweight.

diagram shown in Figure 5.6 suggests that a tree of size 5 should be selected. The optimal tree of this size is shown in Figure 5.7. Here, the first split involves the weight of
the mother. Mothers with weights at last menstrual period below 110 lbs produce
babies with very low birthweights, the average being 2549 g. Mothers of 110 lbs and
above are next split according to whether they had suffered uterine irritability, those

5.4   Summary

The use of tree-based models is perhaps relatively unfamiliar to many statisticians, although researchers in other fields have found trees to be an attractive way to express knowledge and decision-making. In essence, tree growing can be viewed as a family of techniques for adaptive data-driven prediction modelling. Examples of the use of tree models in medicine are to be found in Goldman *et al.* (1982, 1996), Levy *et al.* (1985), McConnochie *et al.* (1993), Choi *et al.* (1991), Temkin *et al.* (1995) and Ciampi *et al.* (2002). The tree approach often gives better insights into the structure than most competing methods, but extensive exploration and careful interpretation are always necessary to arrive at sound conclusions, a sentiment that is true of all exploratory statistical methods. The increasing availability of suitable software such as that described below will hopefully lead to more statisticians considering these methods and uncovering more about both their strengths and their weaknesses.

who had forming a terminal node with average birthweight of 2410 g. Next, women who had not suffered uterine irritability are split into smokers and non-smokers. Finally, the resulting non-smokers are split by race into black/other and white. The final five subgroups are ordered by average birthweight of their babies.

Software

Again, as with GAMs, software for fitting and plotting classification and regression trees is not available in all the major packages. What is available is as follows:

S-PLUS The `tree` function (for fitting both classification and regression trees);
　　　　The `cv.tree` function (for cross-validation in association with `prune.tree`).

(Details on the fitting of tree models using S-PLUS are given in Everitt, 2001b.) The primary tree-related website is http://www.recursive-partitioning.com.

Exercises

5.1 Investigate which variables are needed in a logistic regression model for the response variable *low*.

5.2 Fit a tree model for the response variable *low* which includes only the two categorical variables *smoke* and *race*.

5.3 Construct an optimal classification tree for the prostatic cancer data given in Chapter 1 (Table 1.3). Compare the conclusions you draw from the tree you derive with those given by the logistic regression approach described in Chapter 1.

5.4 The data shown in Table 5.10 relate to air pollution in 41 cities in the USA. The response variable (SO_2) is the annual mean concentration of sulphur dioxide, in micrograms per cubic metre. Investigate using both multiple regression and regression trees which of the six explanatory variables are the most important determinants of pollution.

Table 5.10 Air pollution in US cities

City	SO₂	Temp	Manuf	Pop	Wind	Precip	Days
Phoenix	10	70.3	213	582	6.0	7.05	36
Little Rock	13	61.0	91	132	8.2	48.52	100
San Francisco	12	56.7	453	716	8.7	20.66	67
Denver	17	51.9	454	515	9.0	12.95	86
Hartford	56	49.1	412	158	9.0	43.37	127
Wilmington	36	54.0	80	80	9.0	40.25	114
Washington	29	57.3	434	757	9.3	38.89	111
Jacksonville	14	68.4	136	529	8.8	54.47	116
Miami	10	75.5	207	335	9.0	59.80	128
Atlanta	24	61.5	368	497	9.1	48.34	115
Chicago	110	50.6	3344	3369	10.4	34.44	122
Indianapolis	28	52.3	361	746	9.7	38.74	121
Des Moines	17	49.0	104	201	11.2	30.85	103
Wichita	8	56.6	125	277	12.7	30.58	82
Louisville	30	55.6	291	593	8.3	43.11	123
New Orleans	9	68.3	204	361	8.4	56.77	113
Baltimore	47	55.0	625	905	9.6	41.31	111
Detroit	35	49.9	1064	1513	10.1	30.96	129
Minneapolis	29	43.5	699	744	10.6	25.94	137
Kansas	14	54.5	381	507	10.0	37.00	99
St Louis	56	55.9	775	622	9.5	35.89	105
Omaha	14	51.5	181	347	10.9	30.18	98
Albuquerque	11	56.8	46	244	8.9	7.77	58
Albany	46	47.6	44	116	8.8	33.36	135
Buffalo	11	47.1	391	463	12.4	36.11	166
Cincinnati	23	54.0	462	453	7.1	39.04	132
Cleveland	65	49.7	1007	751	10.9	34.99	155
Columbus	26	51.5	266	540	8.6	37.01	134
Philadelphia	69	54.6	1692	1950	9.6	39.93	115
Pittsburgh	61	50.4	347	520	9.4	36.22	147
Providence	94	50.0	343	179	10.6	42.75	125
Memphis	10	61.6	337	624	9.2	49.10	105
Nashville	18	59.4	275	448	7.9	46.00	119
Dallas	9	66.2	641	844	10.9	35.94	78
Houston	10	68.9	721	1233	10.8	48.19	103
Salt Lake City	28	51.0	137	176	8.7	15.17	89
Norfolk	31	59.3	96	308	10.6	44.68	116
Richmond	26	57.8	197	299	7.6	42.59	115
Seattle	29	51.1	379	531	9.4	38.79	164
Charleston	31	55.2	35	71	6.5	40.75	148
Milwaukee	16	45.7	569	717	11.8	29.07	123

Temp: average annual temperature in °F.
Manuf: number of manufacturing enterprises employing 20 or more workers.
Pop: population size (1970 census); in thousands.
Wind: average windspeed in miles per hour.
Precip: average annual precipitation in inches.
Days: average number of days with precipitation each year.

6

Survival Analysis I: Cox's Regression

6.1   Introduction

In many medical studies, the main outcome variable is the time to the occurrence of a particular event. In a randomized controlled trial of treatment for cancer, for example, surgery, radiation and chemotherapy might be compared with respect to time from randomization and the start of therapy until death. In this case the event of interest is the death of a patient, but in other situations it might be remission from a disease, relief from symptoms, or the recurrence of a particular condition. Such observations are generally referred to by the generic term *survival data*, even when the endpoint or event being considered is not death but something else. Such data generally require special techniques for their analysis for two main reasons:

First, survival data are generally not symmetrically distributed – they will often appear positively skewed, with a few people surviving a very long time compared with the majority; so assuming a normal distribution will not be reasonable.

Second, at the completion of the study, some patients may not have reached the endpoint of interest (death, relapse, etc.). Consequently, the exact survival times are not known. All that is known is that the survival times are greater than the amount of time the individual has been in the study. The survival times of these individuals are said to be *censored* (to be precise, they are right-censored).

When the response variable of interest is a possibly censored survival time, we need special regression techniques for modelling the relationship of the response to explanatory variables of interest. A number of procedures are available, but the most widely used by some margin is that known as *Cox's proportional hazards model*, or *Cox's regression* for short. Introduced by Sir David Cox in 1972 (see Cox, 1972), the method has become one of the most commonly used in medical statistics and the original paper one of the most heavily cited. But again, as with generalized linear models in Chapter 1, an explanation is needed as to why a method introduced three decades ago is making an appearance in a text purporting to be about modern medical statistics. And once again, as in Chapter 1, the explanation I intend to fall back on is that an account of Cox's regression acts as a useful stepping-off point to talk about more recent suggestions for the analysis of survival data. Before describing Cox's model, it may be helpful to remind readers of the two approaches most often used to characterize a set of survival times, namely the *survivor function* and the *hazard function*.

6.2 The survivor function

The survivor function, $S(t)$, is defined as the probability that the survival time, T, is greater than or equal to t, that is,

$$S(t) = \Pr(T > t) \qquad (6.1)$$

A plot of an estimate of $S(t)$ against t is often a useful way of describing the survival experience of a group of individuals. When there are no censored observations in the sample of survival times, a nonparametric estimate of the survivor function is given by

$$\hat{S}(t) = \frac{\text{number of individuals with survival times} \geq t}{\text{number of individuals in the data set}} \qquad (6.2)$$

Because this is simply a proportion, confidence intervals can be obtained for each time t by using the variance estimate

$$\text{Var}(\hat{S}(t)) = \frac{\hat{S}(t)(1 - \hat{S}(t))}{n} \qquad (6.3)$$

where n is the total number of individuals.

Table 6.1 shows survival times of a number of leukaemia patients, along with the values of two other variables which will be ignored here but are needed in exercise 63. There are no censored observations in these data. Figure 6.1 shows the estimated survivor function and its 95% confidence interval. The median survival was 22 weeks, with a 95% confidence interval from 7 to 56 weeks.

A more typical example of survival data, in which censoring occurs, is shown in Table 6.2. These data arise from a randomized, controlled trial to compare two treatments for prostate cancer. (The full data set is given in Andrews and Herzberg, 1985, and the subset of the data shown in Table 6.2 is discussed in Collett, 1994, and

Table 6.1 Survival times of leukaemia patients

WBC	AG	Survival time (weeks)	WBC	AG	Survival time (weeks)
2300	present	65	4400	absent	56
750	present	156	3000	absent	65
4300	present	100	4000	absent	17
2600	present	134	1500	absent	7
6000	present	16	9000	absent	16
10500	present	108	5300	absent	22
10000	present	121	10000	absent	3
17000	present	4	19000	absent	4
5400	present	39	27000	absent	2
7000	present	143	28000	absent	3
9400	present	56	31000	absent	8
32000	present	26	26000	absent	4
35000	present	22	21000	absent	3
100000	present	1	79000	absent	30
100000	present	1	100000	absent	4
52000	present	5	100000	absent	43
100000	present	65			

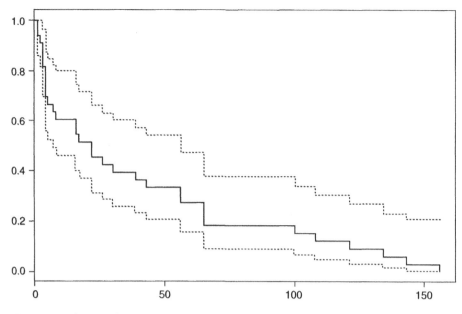

Figure 6.1   Survivor function for leukaemia data with 95% confidence intervals.

Table 6.2   Prostate cancer trial data (Taken with permission of the publisher, CRC Press, from Collett, 1994.)

Treatment	Time	Status	Age	Haem	Size	Gleason
1	65	0	67	13.4	34	8
2	61	0	60	14.4	4	10
2	60	0	77	15.6	3	8
1	58	0	64	16.21	6	9
2	51	0	65	14.1	21	9
1	14	1	73	12.4	18	11
1	43	0	60	13.6	7	9
2	16	0	73	13.8	8	9
1	52	0	73	11.7	5	9
1	59	0	77	12.0	7	10
2	55	0	74	14.3	7	10
2	68	0	71	14.5	19	9
2	51	0	65	14.4	10	9
1	2	0	76	10.7	8	9
1	67	0	70	14.7	7	9
2	66	0	70	16.0	8	9
2	66	0	70	14.5	15	11
2	28	0	75	13.7	19	10
2	50	1	68	12.0	20	11
1	69	1	60	16.1	26	9
1	67	0	71	15.6	8	8
2	65	0	51	11.8	2	6
1	24	0	71	13.7	10	9
2	45	0	72	11.0	4	8

(Continued)

Table 6.2   (*Continued*)

Treatment	Time	Status	Age	Haem	Size	Gleason
2	65	0	51	11.8	2	6
1	24	0	71	13.7	10	9
2	45	0	72	11.0	4	8
2	64	0	74	14.2	4	6
1	61	0	75	13.7	10	12
1	26	1	72	15.3	37	11
1	42	1	57	13.9	24	12
2	57	0	72	14.6	8	10
2	70	0	72	13.8	3	9
2	5	0	74	15.1	3	9
2	54	0	51	15.8	7	8
1	36	1	72	16.4	4	9
2	70	0	71	13.6	2	10
2	67	0	73	13.8	7	8
1	23	0	68	12.5	2	8
1	62	0	63	13.2	3	8

Treatment   1 = placebo, 2 = 1 mg of diethylstilbestrol daily.
Status   1 = dead, 0 = censored.
Time   Survival time in months.
Age   Age at trial entry in years.
Haem   Serum haemoglobin level in g/100 ml.
Size   Size of primary tumour in cm^2.
Gleason   The value of a combined index of tumour stage and grade (the larger the index, the more advanced the tumour).
Source: Andrews and Herzberg (1985).

Everitt and Pickles, 2000.) Patients were randomized to either 1 mg of diethylstilbestrol (DES) or placebo daily by mouth, and their survival was recorded in months. In this section it is only survival in the two treatment groups which is of concern; we shall, however, consider the other variables listed in Table 6.2 later in the chapter.

The simple method used to estimate the survivor function of the data in Table 6.1 cannot now be used for the survival times of patients in the active and placebo groups because of the presence of censored observations. In the presence of censoring, the survivor function is generally estimated using the *Kaplan–Meier estimator*. This method is based on the use of conditional probabilities. For example, suppose that every individual has been followed for 39 days or has died within 39 days so that the proportion of subjects surviving at least 39 days can be computed. After 39 days, some subjects may be lost to follow-up besides those removed from follow-up because of death within 39 days. The proportion of these still followed 39 days who survive day 40 is calculated. The probability of surviving 40 days from study entry equals the probability of surviving day 40 after living 39 days, multiplied by the chance of surviving 39 days (from Harrell, 2001).

The formula for the Kaplan–Meier estimator is as follows:

$$\hat{S}(t) = \prod_{j|t_{(j)} \le t} \left[1 - \frac{d_j}{r_j} \right] \tag{6.3}$$

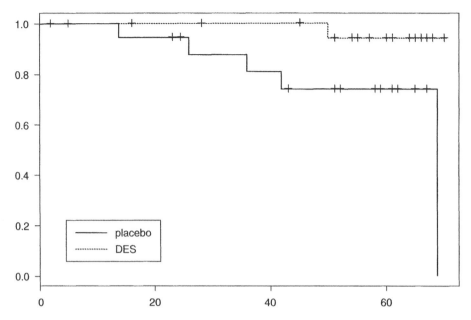

Figure 6.2 Survivor functions for the two treatment groups in the prostate cancer trial.

where $t_{(1)} \leq t_{(2)} \leq \ldots \leq t_{(n)}$ are the ordered survival times, r_j is the number of individuals at risk just before $t_{(j)}$ (including those censored at $t_{(j)}$) and d_j is the number who experience the event of interest (death, etc.) at $t_{(j)}$. So, for example, the survivor function at the second death time, $t_{(2)}$, is equal to the estimated probability of not dying at time $t_{(1)}$ multiplied by the estimated probability of not dying at time $t_{(2)}$, conditional on the individual being still at risk at time $t_{(2)}$. The estimated variance of the Kaplan–Meier estimate of the survivor function is found from

$$\text{Var}(\hat{S}(t)) = [\hat{S}(t)]^2 \sum_{j|t_{(j)} \leq t} \frac{d_j}{r_j(r_j - d_j)} \tag{6.4}$$

Figure 6.2 shows the estimated survivor functions for patients in both the active and placebo groups of the prostate cancer trial (confidence intervals are not given in this case to avoid making the plot look too 'busy'). The data on which the survival curve for the placebo group is based are shown in Table 6.3. A formal test of the equality of the survival curves for the two groups could be made using the *logrank test*. First, the expected number of deaths is computed for each unique death time, or *failure time* (survival time with *Status* = 1), in the data set, assuming that the chances of dying, given that subjects are at risk, are the same for both groups. The total number of expected deaths is then computed for each group by adding the expected number of deaths for each failure time. The test then compares the observed number of deaths in each group with the expected number of deaths using a chi-square test. Full details

Table 6.3 Failure times, number of deaths, number at risk, and number censored in placebo group of prostate cancer trial

j	$t_{(j)}$	d_j	r_j	c_j
1	2	0	18	1
2	14	1	17	0
3	23	0	16	1
4	24	0	15	1
5	26	1	14	0
6	36	1	13	0
7	42	1	12	0
8	43	0	11	1
9	51	0	10	1
10	52	0	9	1
11	58	0	8	1
12	59	0	7	1
13	61	0	6	1
14	62	0	5	1
15	65	0	4	1
16	67	0	3	1
17	69	1	1	0

and formulae are given in Everitt and Rabe-Hesketh (2001). The results of applying the test in this case are:

	N	Observed (O)	Expected (E)	$(O - E)^2/E$
Treatment = 1	18	5	2.47	2.59
Treatment = 2	20	1	3.53	1.81

We thus obtain $X^2 = 4.4$ on 1 degree of freedom, so that $p = 0.036$. There is some evidence of a difference in the survivor functions of the two groups.

Alternative test statistics are available in which the contributions from failure times are differentially weighted – see Everitt and Rabe-Hesketh (2001) for details.

6.3 The hazard function

In the analysis of survival data it is often of interest to assess which periods have high or low chances of death (or whatever the event of interest may be), among those still active at the time. A suitable approach to characterize such risks is the hazard function, $h(t)$, defined as the probability that an individual experiences the event in a small time interval s, given that the individual has survived up to the beginning of the interval, when the size of the time interval approaches zero; mathematically this is written as

$$h(t) = \lim_{s \to 0} \frac{\Pr(t \leq T \leq t + s \,|\, T \geq t)}{s} \quad (6.5)$$

where T is the individual's survival time. The conditioning feature of this definition is very important. For example, the probability of dying at age 100 is very small because

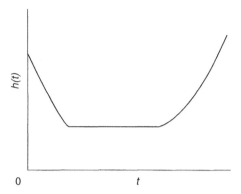

Figure 6.3　Bathtub hazard function.

most people die before that age; in contrast, the probability of a person dying at age 100 who has reached that age is much greater. The hazard function is a measure of how likely an individual is to experience an event as a function of the age of the individual; it is often known as the *instantaneous death rate*.

The hazard function and survivor function are related by the formula

$$S(t) = \exp[-H(t)] \tag{6.6}$$

where $H(t)$ is known as the *integrated hazard* or *cumulative hazard*, and is defined by

$$H(t) = \int_0^t h(u)\mathrm{d}u \tag{6.7}$$

Details of how this relationship arises are given in Everitt and Pickles (2000).

In practice, the hazard function may increase, decrease, remain constant, or have a more complex shape. The hazard function for death in human beings, for example, has the 'bathtub' shape shown in Figure 6.3 It is relatively high immediately after birth, declines rapidly in the early years and then remains approximately constant before beginning to rise again during late middle age.

The hazard function can be estimated as the proportion of individuals experiencing the event of interest in an interval per unit time, given that they have survived to the beginning of the interval, that is,

$$\hat{h}(t) = \frac{d_j}{n_j\left(t_{(j+1)} - t_{(j)}\right)} \tag{6.8}$$

The sampling variation in the estimate of the hazard function within each interval is usually considerable, and so it is rarely plotted directly. Instead the integrated hazard is used. This gives the accumulated risk up until a specific time. Everitt and Rabe-Hesketh (2001) show that this can be estimated as

$$\hat{H}(t) = \sum_j \frac{d_j}{n_j} \tag{6.9}$$

The integrated hazard function for the placebo group in the prostatic cancer trial data is shown in Figure 6.4. The hazard function itself is simply the slope of the cumulative

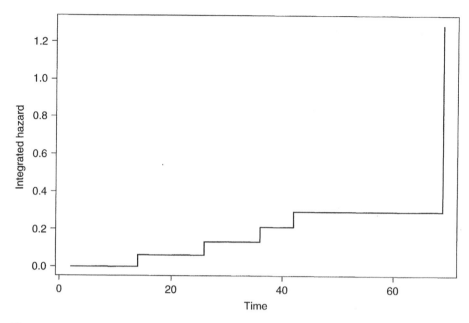

Figure 6.4   Integrated hazard for placebo group in the prostate cancer trial.

hazard. It appears to be approximately constant and then close to zero between 43 and 67 months. However, due to censoring, the risk set (the individuals still alive at the time) decreases from 11 to 1 during that time with only one person at risk at 69 months, explaining the large increase in integrated hazard associated with a single death at 69 months.

6.4   Cox's proportional hazards model

Of most interest in many studies in which survival times are collected is to assess the effects of explanatory variables on these times. The main vehicle for modelling in this case is the hazard function rather than the survivor function, since it does not involve the cumulative history of events. But modelling the hazard function directly as a linear function of explanatory variables is not appropriate since $h(t)$ is restricted to being positive. A more suitable model might be

$$\log h(t) = \beta_0 + \beta_1 x_1 + \cdots + \beta_q x_q \tag{6.10}$$

But this would only be suitable for a hazard function that is constant over time, corresponding to when the distribution of survival times is exponential; such a model is very restrictive since hazards that increase or decrease with time, or have some more complex form, are far more likely to occur in practice. In general, it may be difficult to find the appropriate explicit function of time to include in (6.10). The problem is overcome in the proportional hazards model proposed by Cox (1972), namely

$$\log h(t) = \log h_0(t) + \beta_1 x_1 + \cdots + \beta_q x_q \tag{6.11}$$

where $h_0(t)$ is known as the *baseline hazard function*, being the hazard function for individuals with all explanatory variables equal to zero. This function is left unspecified.

The model can be rewritten as

$$h(t) = h_0(t) \exp(\beta_1 x_1 + \beta_2 x_2 + \cdots + \beta_q x_q) \qquad (6.12)$$

Written in this way, we see that the model forces the hazard ratio between two individuals to be constant over time since

$$\frac{h(t \mid \mathbf{x}_1)}{h(t \mid \mathbf{x}_2)} = \frac{\exp(\boldsymbol{\beta}' \mathbf{x}_1)}{\exp(\boldsymbol{\beta}' \mathbf{x}_2)} \qquad (6.13)$$

where $\mathbf{x}_1$ and $\mathbf{x}_2$ are vectors of covariate values for two individuals and $\boldsymbol{\beta}$ is the vector of regression coefficients. In other words, if an individual has a risk of death at some initial time point that is twice as high as another individual, then at all later times the risk of death remains twice as high. Hence the term 'proportional hazards'. Proportionality of hazards is an assumption that may not necessarily hold. For example, if two individuals with a heart condition receive different treatments, one medical and one surgical, then the individual treated surgically may be at higher risk initially because of the possibility of operative mortality. At a later stage, however, the risk may become the same or even less than for a medically treated individual. In this case, if one of the covariates is a dummy variable indicating whether a person is treated surgically or medically, then the proportional hazards model will not hold. In a given situation the proportionality assumption needs to be checked.

In the Cox model, the baseline hazard describes the common shape of the survival time distribution for all individuals, while the *relative risk function*, $\exp(\boldsymbol{\beta}' \mathbf{x})$, gives the relative level of each individual's hazard. The interpretation of the parameter β_j is that $\exp(\beta_j)$ gives the relative risk change associated with an increase of one unit in x_j, all other explanatory variables remaining constant.

Cox's proportional hazards model is *semi-parametric*; it makes a parametric assumption concerning the effect of the predictors on the hazard function, but makes no assumption regarding the nature of the hazard function itself. In many situations, either the form of the true hazard function is unknown or it is complex and more interest centres on the effects of the predictors than the exact nature of the hazard function – in such situations Cox's method has the distinct advantage of allowing the shape of the hazard function to be ignored.

The Cox model uses only the rank ordering of the failure and censoring times, and the parameters in the model can be estimated by maximizing what is known as a *partial likelihood*. Details are given in Kalbfleisch and Prentice (1980). The partial likelihood is derived by assuming continuous survival times. In reality, however, survival times are measured in discrete units and there are often ties. There are three common methods for dealing with ties, which are described in Kalbfleisch and Prentice (1980).

To illustrate the use of Cox's regression we shall apply it to the data from the trial involving prostate cancer patients given in Table 6.2. To begin, let us fit a Cox model with a single explanatory variable, treatment group. The coefficient of this variable is estimated to be -1.98, with standard error 1.098. The exponentiated coefficient for treatment is 0.14; the hazard in the active treatment group is estimated to be about 14% that in the placebo group. However, the confidence interval for the parameter is found

Table 6.4 Results of applying Cox's regression model to prostate cancer trial data

Covariate	Coef	Std Error	exp(coef)	exp(−coef)	95% CI
Treatment	−1.182	1.210	0.307	3.261	(0.0286, 3.29)
Age	0.044	0.072	1.045	0.957	(0.9074, 1.20)
Haem	−0.022	0.453	0.978	1.022	(0.4027, 2.38)
Size	0.094	0.052	1.099	0.910	(0.9919, 1.22)
Gleason	0.723	0.350	2.061	0.485	(1.0382, 4.09)

Likelihood ratio test = 14.2 on 5 df, $p = 0.0145$.
Wald test = 10.1 on 5 df, $p = 0.0735$.
Score (logrank) test = 15 on 5 df, $p = 0.0104$.

as $(\exp(-1.98 - 1.96 \times 1.098), \exp(-1.98 + 1.96 \times 1.098))$ or $(0.016, 1.19)$, which includes the value one, so there is little evidence of a real treatment effect.

The results from fitting a Cox regression model including all five explanatory variables are shown in Table 6.4. Three tests are reported to judge the joint effect of the five variables, that is, to test the hypothesis that none of the variables is associated with the hazard. The three tests are asymptotically equivalent but differ in finite samples. The likelihood ratio test is generally considered the most reliable, and the Wald test the least (see Therneau and Grambsch, 2000, for reasons). It appears that the Gleason index is most predictive of the hazard function; its exponentiated regression coefficient is 2.061, implying that for each increase in Gleason index by one unit the hazard function approximately doubles, conditional on the remaining explanatory variables remaining constant. But unless one is experienced with using this scale, this is not a particularly helpful statement, since changes of one unit may not be of any practical relevance. More helpful is to refit the model after standardizing the Gleason index to unit variance by dividing by its standard deviation. The standard deviation of the index is 1.34; the hazard function is increased by 2.63 times with an increase in the Gleason index of one standard deviation unit, conditional on the other variables. The associated 95% confidence interval is $(1.05, 6.60)$.

6.5 Left truncation

The Cox model is estimated by maximizing the partial log-likelihood. The partial likelihood is a product of terms, one for each failure time. The subjects contributing to each term are those subjects who are still 'at risk' at the time of the failure; that is, they have not yet died and are still under observation. In the prostate trial, the time scale used in the Cox regression was the time since randomization. An alternative time scale would be age or time since diagnosis. The effect of selecting a different time scale is to change the relative 'alignment' of different people's histories, and this affects the risk sets. For example, suppose a man aged 70 is alive when his father dies at age 95. If the time scale is calendar time, the son would contribute to his father's risk set. However, if the time scale is age, the son does not contribute to his father's risk set if he dies before he is 95.

A person can contribute to a risk set from the time when observation begins. As in the prostate trial, time since observation began is often also the time scale of interest.

Table 6.5   Subset of bone marrow transplant data

Group	Time to platelet recovery (PR)	Status (PR)	Time to death or relapse (DR)	Status (DR)	FAB	Age of donor	Age of patient	MTX
1	13	1	2081	0	0	33	26	0
1	18	1	1602	0	0	37	21	0
1	12	1	1496	0	0	35	26	0
1	13	1	1462	0	0	21	17	0
1	12	1	1433	0	0	36	32	0
1	12	1	1377	0	0	31	22	0
1	17	1	1330	0	0	17	20	0
1	12	1	996	0	0	24	22	0
1	10	1	226	0	0	21	18	0
1	29	1	1199	0	0	40	24	1
1	22	1	1111	0	0	28	19	1
1	34	1	530	0	0	28	17	1
1	22	1	1182	0	0	23	24	1
1	1167	0	1167	0	0	22	27	1
1	21	1	418	1	0	14	18	0
1	16	1	383	1	0	20	15	0
1	21	1	276	1	0	5	18	0
1	20	1	104	1	0	33	20	0
1	26	1	609	1	0	27	27	0
1	37	1	172	1	0	37	40	0

FAB:	French–American–British morphological classification 1 = FAB grade 4 or 5 and AML, 0 = otherwise
MTX:	Methotrexate used as a graft-versus-host-prophylactic or not: 1 = Yes, 0 = No.
PR:	Time to platelet recovery : time in days for platelets to return to normal levels.
Status (PR):	Platelet recovery indicator; 1 – platelets returned to normal levels, 0 = platelets never returned to normal levels.
Time to death:	Time (in days) to death or on study time.
Status (DR):	Death indicator, 1 = dead or relapsed, 0 = alive disease free.
Source:	Klein and Moeschberger (1997).

If the origin of the time scale of interest is earlier than the time when observation began, the data are said to be *left-truncated* because people who experience the event before observation begins are not included in the sample. An example is when the time scale of interest is time since diagnosis but subjects enter the trial some time after diagnosis (*delayed entry*). In order to ensure that the subjects are correctly aligned, we have to specify how long after diagnosis each person entered the trial. Two times are therefore specified per subject; entry time (time when person starts being at risk) and exit time, or event time (time when person dies or is censored), in which both times are measured from the origin of the time scale of interest.

For left-truncated data, we can only model the conditional hazard rates, given that the event time exceeds entry time (otherwise subjects would not be included in the sample). If event time and entry time are conditionally independent given the covariates, then this conditional hazard rate is equivalent to the unconditional hazard rate and no biases are introduced by the left truncation.

As an example of left truncation, we will consider the data given in Table 6.5. These data derive from a multi-centre trial of different preparatory regimens before bone marrow transplant on patients with acute myeloblastic leukaemia (AML) and

Table 6.6 Effect of patient's and donor's age on survival after bone marrow transplant

Covariate	Estimated coefficient	Standard error	Estimate/SE
Age of Patient (P)	−0.810	0.04124	−1.96
Age of Donor (D)	−0.100	0.03717	−2.70
P × D	0.003	0.00114	2.83

acute lymphoblastic leukaemia (ALL), and are discussed in Klein and Moeschberger (1997). Several events post-surgery can change the patient's prognosis for recovery, an important one being the return of platelet count to normal levels. We are interested in disease-free survival since bone marrow transplant (time to death or relapse) in only those patients whose platelet counts have recovered to a self-sustaining level. Although the patients are under observation from the time of the transplant, they start being at risk only after platelet recovery. Entry time is therefore time of platelet recovery (since transplant) and exit time is time of death (since transplant). Potential explanatory variables are disease group (ALL, AML low risk, AML high risk), the age of the patient, the age of the donor, whether methotrexate (MTX) was used as a graft-versus-host prophylactic, and FAB (morphological classification).

Only patients whose platelets recovered (*status (PR)* = 1) are used in the analysis. Initially, we test for the effect of the patient's age and donor's age (both centred at 28 years) and the interaction, giving the estimates shown in Table 6.6. There is significant interaction between the patient's age and the donor's age according to the Wald test. Increasing age of the donor has a positive effect on survival when the patient is 28, with every increase in donor's age being associated with an 8% decrease in the hazard. However, the benefit of donor's age decreases as the patient grows older.

6.6 Extending Cox's model by stratification

In many situations where a Cox model is to be fitted there will be polytomous stratification factors that are either too difficult to model or do not satisfy the proportional hazards assumption. For example, occupation may have a large number of categories and including the possibly dozens of dummy variables needed to model the variable may not be an option when the sample size is only moderate. Another example is a multi-centre trial in which a large number of study sites are involved, and where it is unrealistic to assume common baseline survival curves. In such situations it is possible to use a *stratified Cox model* that allows separate baseline hazards but common coefficients between strata.

As an example we shall return to the bone marrow transplant data and stratify on the use of MTX as a graft-versus-host prophylactic. We repeat the analysis of Klein and Moeschberger (1997) here with covariates group, FAB, and main effects and interaction of age of patient and age of donor. In order to obtain the same estimates as these authors, we use a method of handling ties due to Breslow (1974). The results are given in Table 6.7.

A graph of the predicted survival curves with all covariates equal to their mean values is given in Figure 6.5 Although evaluating predictors at their mean does not make much sense for categorical variables such as group, the graph still gives an impression

Table 6.7   Results from Cox's regression model for bone marrow transplant data stratified on MTX

Covariate	Estimated regression coefficient	Standard error	Estimate/SE
g2	−1.752	0.43761	−4.00
g3	−0.750	0.40769	−1.84
FAB	1.278	0.32494	3.93
Age of patient (P)	0.042	0.02229	1.87
Age of donor (D)	−0.035	0.02068	−1.67
P × D	0.002	0.00122	1.87

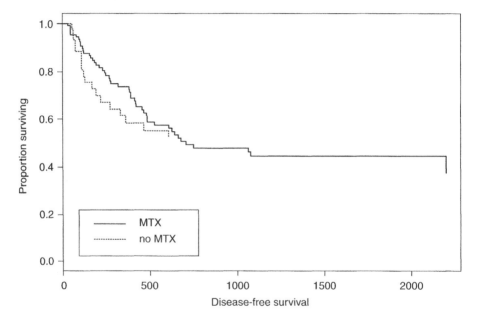

Figure 6.5   Fitted survival curves for bone marrow transplant data where covariates are evaluated at the mean.

of how different the shapes of the survival curves are in the two strata. The difference in survival functions between patients with and without MTX increases early on and then decreases again.

6.7   Checking the specification of a Cox model

Cox's regression model makes two key assumptions. The first of these is that the effect of covariates is additive and linear on a log-hazard scale. This linearity assumption is similar to that found in most other modelling methods we have considered in previous chapters.

The second key assumption is that the ratio of the hazards of two individuals is the same at all times. This proportionality assumption applies to all regressors in the model and not just the treatment effect, and a lack of proportionality can arise for a variety of reasons:

1. Non-instantaneous treatment benefit. A treatment may require some time to be implemented following the randomization time point or may require several sessions to become effective. Some treatments may carry short-term risks which it is hoped are compensated by longer-term benefits. Surgical treatments typically are of this kind, with complications leading to initial excess mortality when compared to a non-surgical treatment.
2. The effect 'wears off' over time. The treatment might halt disease progression only temporarily or the disease may become progressively insensitive to the treatment as the treatment period is extended.
3. A predictor variable may be time-varying but the model represents its effect as due to a single baseline measure. As time goes on, the baseline measure comes to reflect the contemporaneous value of the covariate less and less well and thus becomes less predictive of subsequent survival. For the treatment variable, this can arise through a 'drift' away from the treatment protocol, for example, as a result of increasing non- and poor compliance by patients or inadequate monitoring. For covariate effects such as measures of disease severity, individual variation in the progression of the disease will mean that severity at baseline no longer reflects current severity.
4. Baseline measures are measured subject to error at the time of measurement.
5. Effects are not uniform across patients. This might arise where the treatment benefit applies only to a subsample of individuals, such that over time those for whom treatment has no effect are lost from the treated sample.

To an extent, the particular tests and checks that one might use of the modelling assumptions and the extensions of the model that might be considered, will depend upon which of these possible causes of non-proportionality are suspected. As in the checking of other models, residuals play a key role. A number of different residuals have been proposed for the Cox model.

- *Cox–Snell residual.* This is defined for the ith individual as

$$r_{Ci} = \exp(\hat{\boldsymbol{\beta}}' \mathbf{x}_i) \hat{H}_0(t_i) \tag{6.14}$$

where $\hat{H}_0(t_i)$ is the estimated cumulative baseline hazard function at time t_i, the observed survival time of the individual. If the model is correct, then r_{Ci} will follow an exponential distribution with mean one, regardless of the actual distributional form of $S(t_i)$.
- *Martingale residual.* This is formed by taking the difference between the event indicator, δ_i and the Cox–Snell residual:

$$r_{Mi} = \delta_i - r_{Ci} \tag{6.15}$$

Such residuals can be used to assess whether the survival experience of any particular patients is poorly predicted by the model, with large negative or positive residuals indicating a lack of fit. They can also be used together with continuous covariates for assessing the functional form required for the covariate; a random scatter about zero indicates that the variable does not need transforming.

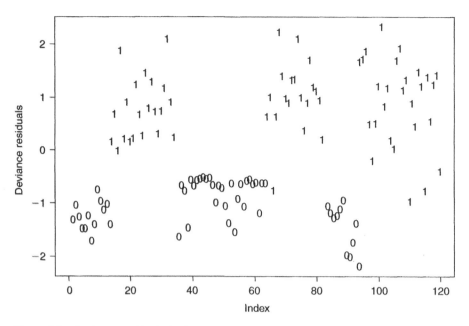

Figure 6.6 Deviance residuals for bone marrow transplant data with censored observations labelled 1 and uncensored labelled 0.

- *Deviance residual.* This may be calculated from the Martingale residual as follows:

$$r_{Di} = \text{sign}\left(r_{Mi}\sqrt{-2[r_{Mi} + \delta_i \ln(\delta_i - r_{Mi})]}\right) \tag{6.16}$$

Such residuals are particularly useful in identifying individuals whose survival is poorly predicted by the model, such individuals being indicated by large negative or positive values of r_{Di}.

- *Schoenfeld or efficient score residual.* Schoenfeld (1982) suggested the use of residuals derived as the first derivative of the partial log-likelihood function with respect to an explanatory variable. For the jth explanatory variable, the residual is defined as

$$r_{Sij} = \frac{x_{ij} - \sum_{r(i)} x_{rj} \exp(\beta' x_r)}{\sum_{r(i)} x_{rj} \exp(\beta' x_r)} \tag{6.17}$$

This residual is large in absolute value if a case's explanatory variable value differs substantially from the explanatory variable values of subjects whose estimated risk of failure is large at the case's time of failure or censoring. The Schoenfeld residual is useful for detecting potentially influential points.

As examples of the use of these plots, Figure 6.6 shows a graph of deviance residuals against the observation number for the bone marrow transplant data with censored and uncensored observations labelled, and Figure 6.7 shows plots of the scaled Schoenfeld residuals against time for each coefficient. In Figure 6.6 none of the

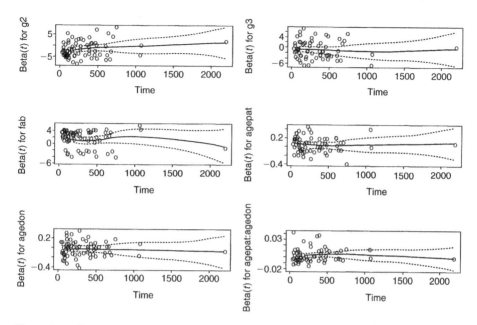

Figure 6.7 Scaled Schoenfeld residuals versus time for all covariates used in the bone marrow transplant data.

deviance residuals is large enough to cause concern. In Figure 6.7 the fitted curves can be interpreted as estimates of $\beta(t)$ if the coefficients were allowed to vary over time. A flat line indicates that the hazards are proportional for different values of the corresponding covariate. The only variable where the assumption may be suspect is FAB.

6.8 Summary

Cox's regression is a widely used technique for investigating the relationship between a response variable which is a (possibly) censored time-to-event variable and a set of explanatory variables of interest. In the next chapter we shall consider some extensions of the model to deal with time-varying covariates and correlated survival times.

Software

Software for survival analysis will be discussed at the end of Chapter 7.

Exercises

6.1 Investigate in more detail which of the five explanatory variables in the prostate cancer data should be retained in a Cox model for the survival times.

6.2 For the final model selected in your answer to Exercise 6.1 check assumptions by using a number of the residuals described in the text.

6.3 In Table 6.1 *WBC* represents the white blood count of a patient and *AG* the presence or absence of a morphological characteristic of the white blood cells.

   (a) Test for a difference in survival between patients with AG = absent and AG = present.

   (b) Plot the integrated hazard functions for both groups as well as the logarithm of the integrated hazard. Are the logarithms of the cumulative hazards parallel?

   (c) Fit a logistic regression model to the data after defining a binary response, survival for at least 24 weeks, and death before 24 weeks. Use both explanatory variables and their interaction. (You may need to rescale WBC.) Compare your results with those observed from applying a Cox proportional hazards model.

6.4 The data below show the survival times in days of two groups of 45 patients suffering from gastric cancer. Group 1 received chemotherapy and radiation; group 2 received only chemotherapy. An asterisk indicates censoring. Plot the Kaplan– Meier survival curves of each group and test for a difference using the logrank test. Show that this is equivalent to fitting a Cox regression model to the data with treatment group as the single covariate.

Group 1			Group 2		
17	185	542	1	383	778
42	193	567	63	383	786
44	195	577	105	388	797
48	197	580	125	394	955
60	208	795	182	408	968
72	234	855	216	460	977
74	235	1174*	250	489	1245
95	254	1214	262	523	1271
103	307	1232*	301	524	1420
108	315	1366	301	535	1460*
122	401	1455*	342	562	1516*
144	445	1585*	354	569	1551
167	464	1622*	356	675	1690*
170	484	1626*	358	676	1694
183	528	1936*	380	748	

7

Survival Analysis II: Time-dependent Covariates, Frailty and Tree Models

7.1 Introduction

In this chapter we consider three further topics related to survival time data, namely, time-dependent covariates, random effects in survival models (frailty) and tree-structured survival analysis. Each of these can provide a valuable additional tool for investigating survival time data in particular circumstances, as we shall try to illustrate.

7.2 Time-dependent covariates

Studies in which survival data are collected often include covariates with values that do not remain fixed over time. Individuals might, for example, have laboratory measurements made repeatedly during the time they were observed. A small hypothetical data set of this kind in shown in Table 7.1.

How can we now fit a Cox regression model that makes allowance for the changes in such variables? In essence it is very simple; the survival period of each individual is divided up into a sequence of shorter survival spells, each characterized by an entry and exit time, and within which covariate values remain fixed. Thus the data for each individual are represented by a number of shorter censored intervals and possibly one

Table 7.1 Hypothetical survival data with a time-varying covariate

Individual	Laboratory measurement (day)			Survival time	Status
	0	60	120		
1	0.5	0.7	0.8	130	1
2	0.2	0.6	0.3	190	1
3	0.2	0.4	–	70	0

Status: 1 = dead, 0 = censored.

Table 7.2   Rearranged data from Table 7.1

Individual	Interval (T_1, T_2)	Lab measurement	Status
1	0,60	0.5	0
1	61,120	0.7	0
1	121,130	0.8	1
2	0,60	0.2	0
2	61,120	0.6	0
2	121,190	0.3	1
3	0,60	0.2	0
3	61,70	0.4	0

The survival time for each interval is calculated as $T_2 - T_1$.

interval ending with the occurrence of the event of interest (death, for example). Table 7.2 shows the data in Table 7.1 rearranged in this way.

It may be thought that the observations in Table 7.2 that arise from the same individual are 'correlated' and so not suitable for Cox's regression as described in the previous chapter. Fortunately this is not an issue, since the partial likelihood on which estimation is based has a term for each unique death or event time, and involves sums over those observations that are available or at risk at the actual event date. Since the intervals for a particular individual do not overlap, the likelihood will involve at most only one of the observations for the individual, and so will still be based on independent observations. The values of the covariates between event times do not enter the partial likelihood. So applying Cox's model to survival data with time-varying covariates is little more complex than for time-fixed covariates.

One circumstance where the use of time-varying covariates may be helpful is where the timing of the delivery of one or both treatments is not under complete experimental control. Such circumstances frequently arise in organ and tissue transplantation, where at the time of randomization no suitably well-matched donors may be available for all patients. Two comparisons then become of interest. The first essentially defines the treatment as that given, that is, a waiting time of unknown duration followed by transplantation, and compares survival over both waiting and post-transplant survival periods combined. The second defines the treatment as transplantation for which only the post-transplant survival is relevant. These correspond to the two rather different clinical circumstances of considering the treatment alternatives of a patient for whom a well-matched donor is already available (the second case) and a patient for whom one is yet to be found (the first case). Without a very rigorous protocol, it is often unreasonable to assume that the waiting time to find a well-matched donor is independent of transplant survival, since matching criteria are likely to be relaxed as the waiting time increases and transplantation may only be possible if the patient is fit enough to survive surgery. Despite this potential difficulty, we shall now illustrate the use of Cox's regression with time-varying covariates with an example of this type, using the well-known set of survival times of potential heart transplant recipients from their date of acceptance into the Stanford heart transplant programme. The data are shown in Table 7.3 in the form described previously. So, for example, patient 3 waited a single day for a transplant and then died after 15 days. In these data patients change treatment status during the course of the study. Specifically, a patient is part of the control group until a suitable donor is located and transplantation takes

Table 7.3   Stanford heart transplant data

ID	Start	Stop	Event	Age	Year	Surgery	Transplant
1	0.0	50.0	1	−17.155	0.123	0	0
2	0.0	6.0	1	3.836	0.255	0	0
3	0.0	1.0	0	6.297	0.266	0	0
3	1.0	16.0	1	6.297	0.266	0	1
4	0.0	36.0	0	−7.737	0.490	0	0
4	36.0	39.0	1	−7.737	0.490	0	1
5	0.0	18.0	1	−27.214	0.608	0	0
6	0.0	3.0	1	6.5955	0.701	0	0
7	0.0	51.0	0	2.8693	0.780	0	1
7	51.0	675.0	1	2.8693	0.780	0	1
8	0.0	40.0	1	−2.650	0.835	0	0
9	0.0	85.0	1	−0.838	0.857	0	0
10	0.0	12.0	1	−5.498	0.862	0	0
10	12.0	58.0	1	−5.498	0.862	0	1
11	0.0	26.0	0	−0.019	0.873	0	0
11	26.0	153.0	1	−0.019	0.873	0	1
12	0.0	8.0	1	5.194	0.964	0	0
13	0.0	17.0	0	6.574	0.969	0	0
13	17.0	81.0	1	6.574	0.969	0	1
14	0.0	37.0	0	6.012	0.972	0	0
14	37.0	1387.0	1	6.012	0.972	0	1
15	0.0	1.0	1	5.815	0.991	1	0
16	0.0	28.0	0	1.448	1.070	0	0
16	28.0	308.0	1	1.448	1.070	0	1
17	0.0	36.0	1	−27.669	1.076	0	0
18	0.0	20.0	0	8.849	1.087	0	0
18	20.0	43.0	1	8.849	1.087	0	1
19	0.0	37.0	1	11.124	1.133	0	0
20	0.0	18.0	0	7.280	1.331	0	0
20	18.0	28.0	1	7.280	1.331	0	1
21	0.0	8.0	0	−4.657	1.339	0	0
21	8.0	1032.0	1	−4.657	1.339	0	1
22	0.0	12.0	0	−5.216	1.462	0	0
22	12.0	51.0	1	−5.216	1.462	0	1
23	0.0	3.0	0	10.357	1.528	0	0
23	3.0	733.0	1	10.357	1.528	0	1
24	0.0	83.0	0	3.800	1.566	0	0
24	83.0	219.0	1	3.800	1.566	0	1
25	0.0	25.0	0	−14.776	1.574	0	0
25	25.0	1800.0	0	−14.776	1.574	0	1
26	0.0	1401.0	0	−17.465	1.582	0	0
27	0.0	263.0	1	−39.214	1.591	0	0
28	0.0	71.0	0	6.023	1.684	0	0
28	71.0	72.0	1	6.023	1.684	0	1
29	0.0	35.0	1	2.434	1.785	0	0
30	0.0	16.0	0	−3.088	1.884	0	0
30	16.0	852.0	1	−3.088	1.884	0	1
31	0.0	16.0	1	6.886	1.895	0	0
32	0.0	17.0	0	16.408	1.911	0	0
32	17.0	77.0	1	16.408	1.911	0	1
33	0.0	51.0	0	0.903	2.157	0	0
33	51.0	1587.0	0	0.903	2.157	0	1
34	0.0	23.0	0	−7.447	2.198	0	0

(Continued)

Table 7.3   (*Continued*)

ID	Start	Stop	Event	Age	Year	Surgery	Transplant
34	23.0	1572.0	0	−7.447	2.199	0	1
35	0.0	12.0	1	−4.534	2.308	0	0
36	0.0	46.0	0	0.925	2.508	0	0
36	46.0	100.0	1	0.925	2.508	0	1
37	0.0	19.0	0	13.500	2.565	0	0
37	19.0	66.0	1	13.500	2.565	0	1
38	0.0	4.5	0	−6.530	2.593	0	0
38	4.5	5.0	1	−6.530	2.593	0	1
39	0.0	2.0	0	2.519	2.634	0	0
39	2.0	53.0	1	2.519	2.634	0	1
40	0.0	41.0	0	0.482	2.648	1	0
40	41.0	1408.0	0	0.482	2.648	1	1
41	0.0	58.0	0	−2.697	2.883	1	0
41	58.0	1322.0	0	−2.697	2.883	1	1
42	0.0	3.0	1	−11.559	2.888	0	0
43	0.0	2.0	1	−4.608	3.058	1	0
44	0.0	40.0	1	−5.421	3.165	1	0
45	0.0	1.0	0	−11.817	3.264	0	0
45	1.0	45.0	1	−11.817	3.264	0	1
46	0.0	2.0	0	0.611	3.277	1	0
46	2.0	996.0	1	0.611	3.277	1	1
47	0.0	21.0	0	−0.901	3.340	0	0
47	21.0	72.0	1	−0.901	3.340	0	1
48	0.0	9.0	1	8.036	3.348	0	0
49	0.0	36.0	0	−11.346	3.376	1	0
49	36.0	1142.0	0	−11.346	3.376	1	1
50	0.0	83.0	0	−2.114	3.376	1	0
50	83.0	980.0	1	−2.114	3.376	1	1
51	0.0	32.0	0	0.734	3.477	0	0
51	32.0	285.0	1	0.734	3.477	0	1
52	0.0	102.0	1	−6.752	3.565	0	0
53	0.0	41.0	0	−0.657	3.751	0	0
53	41.0	188.0	1	−0.657	3.751	0	1
54	0.0	3.0	1	−0.208	3.751	0	0
55	0.0	10.0	0	4.454	3.855	0	0
55	10.0	61.0	1	4.454	3.855	0	1
56	0.0	67.0	0	−9.257	3.923	0	0
56	67.0	942.0	0	−9.257	3.923	0	1
57	0.0	149.0	1	−6.735	3.951	0	0
58	0.0	21.0	0	0.016	3.978	1	0
58	21.0	343.0	1	0.016	3.978	1	1
59	0.0	78.0	0	−6.617	3.995	1	0
59	78.0	916.0	0	−6.617	3.995	1	1
60	0.0	3.0	0	1.054	4.131	0	0
60	3.0	68.0	1	1.054	4.131	0	1
61	0.0	2.0	1	4.564	4.175	0	0
62	0.0	69.0	1	−8.646	4.189	0	0
63	0.0	27.0	0	−15.340	4.197	0	0
63	27.0	842.0	0	−15.340	4.197	0	1
64	0.0	33.0	0	0.816	4.337	1	0
64	33.0	584.0	1	0.816	4.337	1	1
65	0.0	12.0	0	3.294	4.430	0	0
65	12.0	78.0	1	3.294	4.430	0	1
66	0.0	32.0	1	5.213	4.468	0	0

(*Continued*)

Table 7.3   (*Continued*)

ID	Start	Stop	Event	Age	Year	Surgery	Transplant
67	0.0	57.0	0	−28.449	4.476	0	0
67	57.0	285.0	1	−28.449	4.476	0	1
68	0.0	3.0	0	−2.760	4.517	0	0
68	3.0	68.0	1	−2.760	4.517	0	1
69	0.0	10.0	0	−0.011	4.668	0	0
69	10.0	670.0	0	−0.011	4.668	0	1
70	0.0	5.0	0	5.002	4.712	0	0
70	5.0	30.0	1	5.002	4.712	0	1
71	0.0	31.0	0	−0.591	4.805	0	0
71	31.0	620.0	0	−0.591	4.805	0	1
72	0.0	4.0	0	−21.273	4.871	0	0
72	4.0	596.0	0	−21.273	4.871	0	1
73	0.0	27.0	0	8.331	4.947	0	0
73	27.0	90.0	1	8.331	4.947	0	1
74	0.0	5.0	0	−18.834	4.966	0	0
74	5.0	17.0	1	−18.834	4.966	0	1
75	0.0	2.0	1	4.181	4.997	0	0
76	0.0	46.0	0	4.085	5.010	1	0
76	46.0	545.0	0	4.085	5.010	1	1
77	0.0	21.0	1	−6.888	5.016	0	0
78	0.0	210.0	0	0.704	5.092	0	0
78	210.0	515.0	0	0.704	5.092	0	1
79	0.0	67.0	0	5.782	5.166	0	0
79	67.0	96.0	1	5.782	5.166	0	1
80	0.0	26.0	0	−1.555	5.183	1	0
80	26.0	482.0	0	−1.555	5.183	1	1
81	0.0	6.0	0	4.893	5.284	0	0
81	6.0	445.0	0	4.893	5.284	0	1
82	0.0	428.0	0	−18.798	4.085	0	0
83	0.0	32.0	0	5.309	5.317	0	0
83	32.0	80.0	1	5.309	5.317	0	1
84	0.0	37.0	0	−5.281	5.333	0	0
84	37.0	334.0	1	−5.281	5.333	0	1
85	0.0	5.0	1	−0.019	5.352	0	0
86	0.0	8.0	0	0.920	5.415	0	0
86	8.0	397.0	0	0.920	5.415	0	1
87	0.0	60.0	0	−1.747	5.470	0	0
87	60.0	110.0	1	−1.747	5.470	0	1
88	0.0	31.0	0	6.363	5.489	0	0
88	31.0	370.0	0	6.363	5.489	0	1
89	0.0	139.0	0	3.047	5.511	0	0
89	139.0	207.0	1	3.047	5.511	0	1
90	0.0	160.0	0	4.033	5.514	1	0
90	160.0	186.0	1	4.033	5.514	1	1
91	0.0	340.0	1	−0.405	5.533	0	0
92	0.0	310.0	0	−3.017	5.572	0	0
92	310.0	340.0	0	−3.017	5.572	0	1
93	0.0	28.0	0	−0.249	5.777	0	0
93	28.0	265.0	0	−0.249	5.777	0	1
94	0.0	4.0	0	−4.159	5.955	1	0
94	4.0	165.0	1	−4.158	5.955	1	1
95	0.0	2.0	0	−7.718	5.977	0	0
95	2.0	16.0	1	−7.718	5.977	0	1
96	0.0	13.0	0	−21.350	6.010	0	0

(*Continued*)

Table 7.3   (*Continued*)

ID	Start	Stop	Event	Age	Year	Surgery	Transplant
96	13.0	180.0	0	−21.350	6.010	0	1
97	0.0	21.0	0	−24.383	6.144	0	0
97	21.0	131.0	0	−24.383	6.144	0	1
98	0.0	96.0	0	−19.370	6.204	0	0
98	96.0	109.0	0	−19.370	6.204	0	1
99	0.0	21.0	1	1.834	6.234	0	0
100	0.0	38.0	0	−12.939	6.396	1	0
100	38.0	39.0	0	−12.939	6.396	1	1
101	0.0	31.0	0	1.517	6.418	0	0
102	0.0	11.0	0	−7.608	6.472	0	0
103	0.0	6.0	1	−8.684	−0.049	0	0

Surgery: 0 = no previous surgery, 1 = previous surgery.
Transplant: 0 = no transplant, 1 = transplant.
Event: 0 = censored, 1 = died.

place, at which time he joins the treatment group. So treatment is a time-dependent covariate. The other covariates to be considered are age (in years minus 48), whether the patient had had previous heart surgery, and waiting time for acceptance into the programme (years since 1 October 1967).

The results of fitting a number of proportional hazards models to these data are shown in Table 7.4. Using the single covariate, *Transplant*, the results of the likelihood ratio test, the Wald test and the logrank test are all the same. There is no evidence that transplantation affects the hazard function.

Including all four covariates, *Transplant*, *Surgery*, *Age* and *Year*, in a Cox model leads to highly significant values for all three test criteria. Clearly not all the covariates have zero regression coefficients. It appears that both age and year are associated with survival.

The last model for which the results appear in Table 7.4 is one which includes *Surgery*, *Age*, *Year*, *Transplant* and a *Year* × *Transplant* interaction. From this model it appears that survival time depends on the time of acceptance into the study; as this increases, the hazard function for the death of a patient decreases. But this claim becomes less clear-cut if we examine the Transplant × time of acceptance interaction which approaches significance, with an effect which is in the opposite direction. According to Kalbfleisch and Prentice (1980), taken together these results imply that the overall quality of patient being admitted to the study is improving with time (possibly due to the relaxation of admission requirements or to improving patient management); but the survival time of the transplanted patients is not improving at the same rate.

A further model which might be considered is one which allows separate baseline hazards for the post-transplanted and pre- or not-transplanted patients, but common coefficients in each group. The results of fitting a particular stratified Cox method of this type are shown in Table 7.5. Plotting the graph of the predicted survival curves in each stratum, with all covariates equal to their mean values (see Figure 7.1), demonstrates the longer survival experience of patients who have a transplant.

As this example illustrates, time-varying covariates can be introduced into a Cox model for survival data very simply. But this apparent simplicity should not disguise the potential problems, the main one being that the inclusion of such covariates runs the risk of biasing the estimated treatment effect if they themselves reflect the

Table 7.4 Results of applying Cox's regression to Stanford Heart Transplant Data

(a) *Transplant* as a single covariate

Covariate	Estimated regression coefficient	Standard error	exp(coef)	exp(−coef)	95% CI for relative risk
Transplant	−0.107	0.127	0.898	1.11	(0.7, 1.15)

Likelihood ratio test = 0.7 on 1 df, $p = 0.400$.
Wald test = 0.7 on 1 df, $p = 0.400$.
Score (logrank) test = 0.7 on 1 df, $p = 0.400$.

(b) Main effects model

Covariate	Estimated regression coefficient	Standard error	exp(coef)	exp(−coef)	95% CI for relative risk
Transplant	−0.142	0.132	0.868	1.152	(0.671, 1.123)
Surgery	−0.664	0.366	0.515	1.943	(0.251, 1.055)
Age	0.028	0.014	1.029	0.972	(1.001, 1.057)
Year	−0.152	0.071	0.859	1.165	(0.748, 0.986)

Likelihood ratio test = 16.8 on 4 df, $p = 0.002$.
Wald test = 16.0 on 4 df, $p = 0.003$.
Score (logrank) test = 16.6 on 4 df, $p = 0.002$.

(c) Main effects plus Transplant × Year interaction

Covariate	Estimated regression coefficient	Standard error	exp(coef)	exp(−coef)	95% CI for relative risk
Surgery	−0.689	0.3671	0.502	1.992	(0.244, 1.031)
Age	0.031	0.0139	1.031	0.970	(1.004, 1.060)
Transplant	−0.430	0.2468	0.650	1.538	(0.401, 1.055)
Year	−0.160	0.0716	0.852	1.174	(0.741, 0.981)
Transplant × Year	0.096	0.6983	1.101	0.909	(0.960, 1.262)

Likelihood ratio test = 18.76 on 5 df, $p = 0.0021$.
Wald test = 18.38 on 5 df, $p = 0.0025$.
Score (logrank) test = 19.26 on 5 df, $p = 0.0017$.

Table 7.5 Stratified Cox's model results for heart transplant data

Covariate	Estimated regression coefficient	Standard error	exp(coef)	exp(−coef)	95% CI
Surgery	−0.651	0.369	0.5213	1.918	(0.253, 1.075)
Age	0.028	0.014	1.0288	0.972	(1.001, 1.057)
Year	−0.157	0.071	0.8543	1.171	(0.743, 0.982)

Likelihood ratio test = 16.27 on 3 df, $p = 0.001$.
Wald test = 15.45 on 3 df, $p = 0.001$.
Score (logrank) test = 16.11 on 3 df, $p = 0.001$.

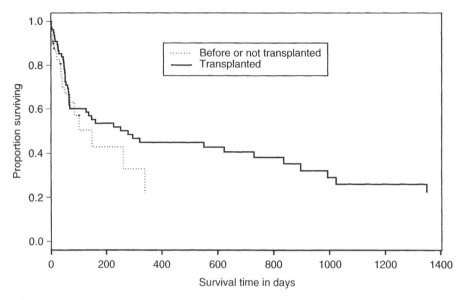

Figure 7.1   Predicted survival curves for heart transplant data.

development of the disease process and so may be partly influenced by treatment. Biochemical or physical measures of disease are obvious examples. This is well illustrated in an example given by Altman and DeStavola (1994). High levels of bilirubin and low levels of albumin reflect advanced biliary cirrhosis and are highly prognostic. A treatment that improves cirrhosis will tend to reduce bilirubin levels and increase those of albumin. Altman and DeStavola showed how much of the significant and substantial estimate of treatment effect could be removed by the inclusion into the model of updated values of either of these variables. From the point of view of treatment effect estimation, updating these variables is most unwise, casting unnecessary doubt on treatment differences. From the point of view of a scientific investigation of the development of the process and for constructing prognostic indices, their inclusion will be of more interest.

Thus, it is important that *internal* or *endogenous* variables should be distinguished from *external* or *exogenous* variables. External variables are either predetermined, as in the case of a patient's age, or vary independently of survival, for instance the weather. However, for many time-varying variables their status as internal or external is uncertain, which explains our caution. It is perhaps most helpful to think of internal variables as being those that are 'causally downstream' of treatment, but the link between treatment and the internal variable does not have to be a direct one. Thus if the poor health of those on the worse or placebo treatment results in their choosing to move to a more pleasant and health-promoting climate, then not even the weather is external!

7.3   Random effects models for survival data

Cox's proportional hazards model, as described in the previous chapter, has become the workhorse of regression analysis for censored time-to-event data. But one of the implicit assumptions of the method, namely that the survival times observed are independent of one another, is not necessarily valid in all situations in which survival times are collected. Some types of studies generate *correlated* survival times, and a suitable model must account for the correlations. Some examples of such studies are:

- survival times of individuals who have been formed into matched groups similar on a set of prognostically relevant variables;
- survival times of individuals related by, for example, family membership, marriage, exposure to some agent (assuming this is not a predictor in the model), etc.;
- recurrent or repeated events, where the same event, for example myocardial infarction, can happen several times for an individual.

The most common way of dealing with correlated survival time data is to use an approach analogous to the random effects models described in Chapter 2. Random effects are again used to generate the likely dependence between the observations, and, conditional on the random effects, the observations are assumed independent. For survival data, the random effects are built into a Cox model for the data, and are also given a special name, *frailty*, a term first introduced by Vaupel *et al.* (1979).

Frailty models can be fitted to survival or other time-to-event data by what is known as a *penalized partial likelihood* approach, details of which are given in Therneau and Grambsch (2000). As a first illustration of the use of such models, we shall apply one to the data shown in Table 7.6. These data were originally given in Frierich *et al.* (1963) and showed the survival times of pairs of patients with leukaemia when treated with either 6-mercaptopurine (6 MP) or placebo; one member of a pair received the active treatment and one the placebo.

The model that we shall fit to these data is as follows:

$$\log[h_{i(j)}(t)] = \log[h_0(t)] + \beta_1 \text{treatment}_{i(j)} + u_{(j)} \qquad (7.1)$$

where $h_{i(j)}(t)$ is the hazard function of patient i in pair j, $i = 1, 2, j = 1, \ldots, 21$, treatment$_{i(j)}$ is a dummy variable defining which treatment the patient had and $u_{(j)}$ is the random effect, or frailty, associated with pair j. We will assume that the frailties are normally distributed with mean zero and variance σ^2. The results of fitting the model in (7.1) and the usual Cox model to all 42 survival times, ignoring the pairing, are shown in Table 7.7. Here we see that there is very little difference in the two sets of results. This suggests that the pairs of patients were not particularly well matched on the basis of the factors used, or that these factors were of little prognostic significance. The treatment effect is highly significant, with longer survival in the group given 6 MP.

As a further example of dealing with correlated time-to-event data, we shall apply a frailty model to the observations in Table 7.8, which are recurrence times to infection at point of insertion of the catheter for kidney patients using portable dialysis equipment. For each patient two such recurrence times are given. The covariates of interest are age, gender and the presence/absence of disease types GN, ANN and PKD. Here the inclusion of the frailty term in a Cox model allows for the possible correlation between the recurrence times of an individual.

The results of applying both the usual Cox's regression model and the shared frailty model to these data are shown in Table 7.9. The results are again fairly similar, except for the covariate *pkd*, which is estimated to have a significant effect in the former but is non-significant in the latter. For both models *sex* is estimated to have greatest effect on the hazard function. In the frailty model, for example, the hazard for women is estimated to be between 6% and 40% that for men.

Table 7.6   Survival times of pairs of leukaemia patients, receiving 6MP or placebo

Survival time	Status	Treatment	Pair
1	1	1	1
1	1	1	2
2	1	1	3
2	1	1	4
3	1	1	5
4	1	1	6
4	1	1	7
5	1	1	8
5	1	1	9
8	1	1	10
8	1	1	11
8	1	1	12
8	1	1	13
11	1	1	14
11	1	1	15
12	1	1	16
12	1	1	17
15	1	1	18
17	1	1	19
22	1	1	20
23	1	1	21
6	1	0	19
6	1	0	18
6	1	0	8
6	0	0	1
7	1	0	20
9	0	0	6
10	1	0	2
10	0	0	10
11	0	0	3
13	1	0	14
16	1	0	4
17	0	0	11
19	0	0	7
20	0	0	9
22	1	0	12
23	1	0	16
25	0	0	17
32	0	0	5
34	0	0	15
35	0	0	21

Status: 1 = dead, 0 = censored.
Treatment: 1 = placebo, 0 = 6MP.
Source: Frierich *et al*. (1963).

7.4   Tree-structured survival analysis

In Chapter 5 we described the use of tree models for exploring the relationship between a continuous response variable and a set of explanatory variables. Such models are also useful in the analysis of other types of response, and in this section we shall look briefly at how they can be applied to survival data.

Table 7.7 Results of fitting Cox's model and frailty model to data in Table 7.6

(a) Cox's model

Covariate	Estimated regression coefficient	Standard error	exp(coef)	exp(−coef)	95% CI
Treatment	1.572	0.4124	4.817	0.208	(2.147, 10.81)

Likelihood ratio test = 16.35 on 1 df, $p < 0.0001$.
Wald test = 14.53 on 1 df, $p = 0.0001$.
Score (logrank) test = 17.25 on 1 df, $p < 0.0001$.

(b) Frailty model

Covariate	Estimated regression coefficient	Standard error	exp(coef)	exp(−coef)	95% CI
Treatment	1.574	0.4127	4.826	0.207	(2.149, 10.84)

Likelihood ratio test = 16.48 on 1.07 df, $p < 0.0001$.
Wald test = 14.55 on 1.07 df, $p = 0.0002$.

Table 7.8 Recurrence times for catheter infection in kidney patients

Subject	Time	Status	Age	Sex	Disease
1	8	1	28	1	3
1	16	1	28	1	3
2	23	1	48	2	0
2	13	0	48	2	0
3	22	1	32	1	3
3	28	1	32	1	3
4	447	1	31	2	3
4	318	1	32	2	3
5	30	1	10	1	3
5	12	1	10	1	3
6	24	1	16	2	3
6	245	1	17	2	3
7	7	1	51	1	0
7	9	1	51	1	0
8	511	1	55	2	0
8	30	1	56	2	0
9	53	1	69	2	1
9	196	1	69	2	1
10	15	1	51	1	0
10	154	1	52	1	0
11	7	1	44	2	1
11	333	1	44	2	1
12	141	1	34	2	3
12	8	0	34	2	3
13	96	1	35	2	1
13	38	1	35	2	1

(*Continued*)

Table 7.8   (*Continued*)

Subject	Time	Status	Age	Sex	Disease
14	149	0	42	2	1
14	70	0	42	2	1
15	536	1	17	2	3
15	25	0	17	2	3
16	17	1	60	1	1
16	4	0	60	1	1
17	185	1	60	2	3
17	177	1	60	2	3
18	292	1	43	2	3
18	114	1	44	2	3
19	22	0	53	2	0
19	159	0	53	2	0
20	15	0	44	2	3
20	108	0	44	2	3
21	152	1	46	1	2
21	562	1	47	1	2
22	402	1	30	2	3
22	24	0	30	2	3
23	13	1	62	2	1
23	66	1	63	2	1
24	39	1	42	2	1
24	46	0	43	2	1
25	12	1	43	1	1
25	40	1	43	1	1
26	113	0	57	2	1
26	201	1	58	2	1
27	132	1	10	2	0
27	156	1	10	2	0
28	34	1	52	2	1
28	30	1	52	2	1
29	2	1	53	1	0
29	25	1	53	1	0
30	130	1	54	2	0
30	26	1	54	2	0
31	27	1	56	2	1
31	58	1	56	2	1
32	5	0	50	2	1
32	43	1	51	2	1
33	152	1	57	2	2
33	30	1	57	2	2
34	190	1	44	2	0
34	5	0	45	2	0
35	119	1	22	2	3
35	8	1	22	2	3
36	54	0	42	2	3
36	16	0	42	2	3
37	6	0	52	2	2
37	78	1	52	2	2
29	63	1	60	1	2
38	8	0	60	1	2

Time: recurrence time in days.
Status: 1 = infection occurs, 0 = censored.
Disease: 0 = GN, 1 = AN, 2 = PKD, 3 = other.
Sex: 1 = male, 2 = female.

Table 7.9   Results of fitting Cox's model and frailty model to data in Table 7.9

(a) Cox's model, $n = 76$

Covariate	Estimated regression coefficient	Standard error	exp(coef)	exp(−coef)	95% CI
age	0.002	0.011	1.002	0.998	(0.980, 1.024)
sex	−1.530	0.361	0.217	4.620	(0.107, 0.439)
gn	0.154	0.446	1.166	0.858	(0.520, 2.613)
an	0.440	0.406	1.552	0.644	(0.701, 3.437)
pkd	−1.402	0.636	0.246	4.063	(0.071, 0.857)

Likelihood ratio test = 18.74 on 5 df, $p = 0.0021$.
Wald test   = 21.2 on 5 df, $p = 0.0007$.
Score (logrank) test = 21.52 on 5 df, $p = 0.0006$.

(b) Frailty model

Covariate	Estimated regression coefficient	Standard error	exp(coef)	exp(−coef)	95% CI
age	0.003	0.016	1.003	0.997	(0.972, 1.0345)
sex	−1.806	0.484	0.164	6.089	(0.064, 0.424)
gn	0.295	0.579	1.343	0.745	(0.431, 4.181)
an	0.539	0.582	1.714	0.584	(0.548, 5.364)
pkd	−1.026	0.867	0.358	2.791	(0.066, 1.959)

Variance of random effect = 0.6073.
$R^2 = 0.503$ (max possible = 0.992).
Likelihood ratio test   = 53.07 on 15.91 df, $p < 0.0001$.
Wald test   = 15.58 on 15.91 df, $p = 0.4764$.

The main difference in growing tree models for survival data and for a continuous variable as described in Chapter 5 are:

- the sum-of-squares function used to develop the tree is not suitable for censored survival times;
- the mean value of the response for those observations in a terminal node is not a suitable summary for survival data.

Segal (1998) considers both these problems and suggests that the splitting function for right-censored survival data should be based on maximizing one of the statistics routinely used for testing the equality of the survival distributions of two groups. The most commonly used of these is the logrank test described in the previous chapter, but other possibilities are available that are described in Tarone and Ware (1977) and Harrington and Fleming (1982). And for summarizing the terminal nodes of survival trees, Segal suggests using Kaplan–Meier survival curves.

To illustrate the application of survival trees we shall describe the study reported in Segal (1998), concerned with breast cancer screening and associated risk factors. A cohort of 2089 white women aged between 30 and 79, living in the San Francisco Bay area, who were neither pregnant nor lactating, and who were free of breast cancer, were recruited between 1973 and 1980. Nipple aspirates of breast fluid were collected using a modified breast pump (Petrakis *et al.*, 1981). Each breast fluid specimen was cyto-logically classified according to the most severe epithelial change present (King *et al.*, 1983). This yielded an ordered categorical variable with the following levels: $0 \equiv$ no breast fluid; $1 \equiv$ unsatisfactory specimen; $2 \equiv$ normal specimen; $3 \equiv$ hyperplasia; $4 \equiv$ hyperplasia and atypia; $5 \equiv$ severe atypia. It is important to note that the coding of levels for such ordered categorical covariates is immaterial for tree methods: tree topologies (that is, split variables and associated cut-points) are invariant to mono-tone transformations of the covariates. Cohort follow-up occurred between June 1988 and April 1991. Details on ascertainment and incident breast cancer validation are given by Wrensch *et al.* (1992). The survival time of interest is time to breast cancer from enrolment.

Here we analyse data provided by all women. By not restricting to the subset of parous women we can examine parity (nulli/parous) as a covariate but are precluded from using variables such as age at first pregnancy and breastfeeding. Other covariates included in the tree-structured survival analysis were age (continuous), menopausal status (pre/post), family (mother/sister/daughter) history of breast cancer (yes/no), age at menarche (four ordered levels), education (three ordered levels), place of examin-ation (UCSF/other), and Quetelet's index (continuous). Further variable and cohort information, as well as results from Cox proportional hazards modelling, is provided by Wrensch *et al.* (1992). Excluding cases with missing data reduced the sample to 1639 women. The ability to utilize cases with missing covariate information is one of the strengths of the classification and regression tree approach.

Survival tree results are depicted in Figures 7.2 and 7.3. The top panel of Figure 7.2 displays the large tree prior to pruning. This tree was grown using the logrank statis-tic as the split function, although very similar topologies result from using other two-sample censored data rank statistics. Two additional user-specified parameters control the extent of the tree: the first specifies the minimum node size required in order to entertain splitting (here 30) and the second specifies the minimum proportion of uncensored observations within a node required in order to entertain splitting. This was set at 3%, less than the overall uncensored rate of 4.2%. As described, these settings are not critical provided that a suitably large tree results.

Above each non-terminal node number the covariate and cut-point defining the split are given. Thus, node 1 is split on age with those women aged below 45.5 assigned to node 2 and those aged above 45.5 assigned to node 3. Age was given in (integer) years, so this is unambiguous. Below each terminal node is a summary ratio of num-ber of events (breast cancers) to number of subjects in that node. For example, node 2 consists of the 847 women aged below 45.5 of whom 17 were diagnosed with breast cancer during follow-up. The anticipated low event rate (2%) explains why this large node is not further subdivided, in contrast with the older women for whom the event rate is 6.6%. The Kaplan–Meier survival curves associated with this age split are given in the bottom panel of Figure 7.3.

The bottom panel of Figure 7.2 displays subtree maximal split (logrank) statistics plotted against subtree size (number of terminal nodes) and indexed by subtree root. As discussed, the characteristic 'elbow' is evident. Selection of a pruned tree at or just beyond the elbow is recommended. Interactive pruning based on this plot yields a selected tree as displayed in the top panel of Figure 7.3.

The node 3 older (>45.5) women resulting from the age split described above are further subdivided on the basis of cytology. The cut-point of 2.5 means that those

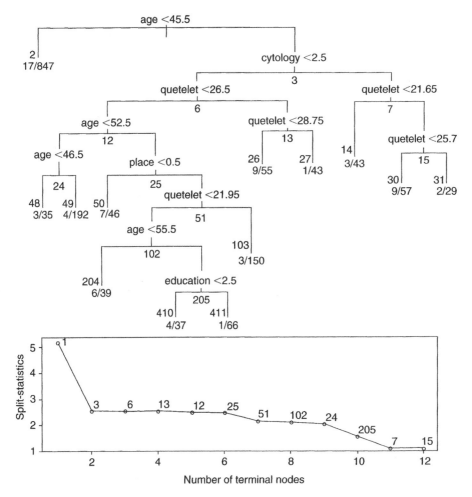

Figure 7.2   Upper panel: survival tree for the breast cancer cohort study grown using all covariates and the logrank split statistic. Lower panel: plot of maximal subtree split statistics tree size (the number of terminal nodes). (Taken with permission from Segal, 1998.)

women who have (favourable) cytological findings (levels 0, 1 and 2) are separated from those with abnormal cytological findings (levels 3, 4 and 5). We anticipate that this latter subgroup of older women with abnormal cytology (node 7) would constitute the prognostic subgroup with poorest survival. However, the older women with normal cytological findings (node 6) are further split on the basis of Quetelet's index, a measure of obesity. Examining the survival curves given in Figure 7.4, it appears that the more obese subgroup (node 13) have comparable survival with the older women with abnormal cytology. Thus, in addition to eliciting an anticipated prognostic subgroup with poor survival, the exploratory survival tree analysis has identified another prognostic subgroup with similarly high risk. (This account is taken directly from Segal, 1998, with permission of the author.)

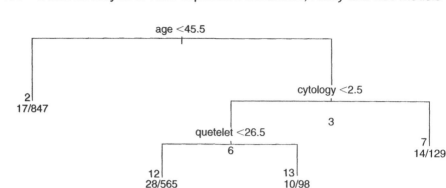

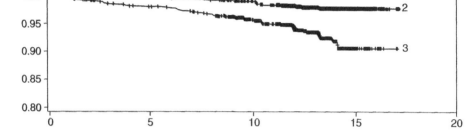

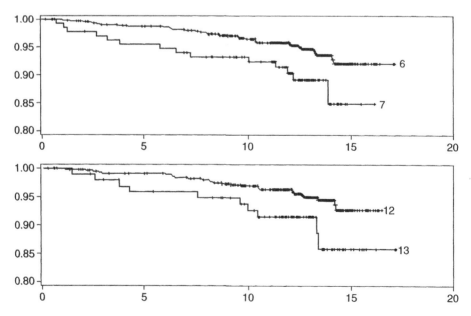

Figure 7.3   Upper panel: pruned tree obtained from initial large tree. Lower panel: Kaplan–Meier curves corresponding to the first split on age with cut point 45.5 years. (Taken with permission from Segal, 1998.)

Figure 7.4   Upper panel: Kaplan–Meier curves corresponding to the second split on cytology finding with cut-point 2.5. Lower panel: Kaplan–Meier curves corresponding to the blind split on Quelelet's index with cut-point 26.5. (Taken with permission from Segal, 1998.)

7.5 Summary

Time-varying covariates can be handled relatively easily in the Cox proportional hazards model, although care is needed to ensure that it is sensible to include such covariates in the modelling process. Correlated survival times can be dealt with by introducing random effects (frailties) into the model. A tree regression approach using splits based on, say, the logrank statistic provides a useful additional tool for analysing survival data.

Software

Survival analysis procedures are readily available in all major software packages:

SAS	`proc lifetest` (for estimating survival curves and testing for differences); `proc phreg` (for fitting proportional hazard models).
STATA	`stcox` command (for fitting Cox's regression model).
S-PLUS	coxph function (for Cox's regression).

Details on the use of SAS, STATA and S-PLUS for survival analysis are given in Der and Everitt (2001), Rabe-Hesketh and Everitt (2000), Everitt (2001b) and Everitt and Rabe-Hesketh (2001).

For tree models in survival analysis, see http://lib.stat.cmu.edu/s/rpart2.

Exercises

7.1 Investigate the heart transplant data further using Cox regression models with interactions. Use some of the diagnostics outlined in Chapter 6 to check the assumptions of the model.

7.2 Reanalyse the kidney infection data to investigate the possibility that interactions are needed in any suitable Cox regression model.

7.3 The data given below arise from a study of prognostic variables in advanced cancer patients. The variables in the data set are:

1 – enrolling institution;
2 – survival time;
3 – status: 1 = alive, 2 = dead;
4 – age;
5 – sex: 1 = male, 2 = female;
6 – calories consumed at meals;
7 – weight loss in last six months.

Fit the following three Cox's regression models to the data:

(a) model with age, sex, calories and weight as covariates;
(b) model with age, sex, calories, weight and institution as covariates;
(c) frailty model for institutions with age, sex, calories and weight as covariates.

Compare results and comment on which model you feel is preferable. Would your comments change if there were 50 enrolling institutions?

1	2	3	4	5	6	7
1	306	2	74	1	1175	12
1	455	2	68	1	1225	15
1	1010	1	56	1	1150	15
2	12	2	74	1	35	−20
2	731	2	64	2	1175	15
2	246	2	58	1	1175	7
2	345	2	64	2	1075	−3
2	93	2	74	1	1225	24
3	310	2	68	2	384	10
3	166	2	61	1	271	34
3	533	2	48	1	388	−11
3	583	2	68	1	1025	7
3	95	2	76	2	625	−24
3	92	2	50	1	1075	13
3	413	1	64	1	413	16

8

Bayesian Methods and Meta-analysis

8.1 Introduction

In this chapter we shall look at two topics in which there have been major advances in the last two decades, namely *Bayesian analysis* and *meta-analysis*. Both are of considerable importance in medicine. In a Bayesian analysis prior information about parameters of interest is incorporated into the model fitting process, and in meta-analysis information from previous studies is integrated so as to provide a more accurate estimate and a more powerful inference about a parameter.

8.2 Bayesian methods

The traditional frequentist approach to a medical investigation is to regard it as if it were entirely novel, and potentially decisive in itself in regard to a particular question or questions of interest. The numerical procedures employed are not formulated to reflect the possibility of progressive learning. By contrast, the focus of Bayesian methods is one of progressive refinement of opinion as data from similar studies and investigations accumulate. This is illustrated in Figure 8.1 in the context of a clinical trial. Knowledge available prior to the current trial is synthesized and formally represented as a probability distribution for the parameter or parameters of interest; this is called the *prior distribution*. The trial is then undertaken and relevant data collected. Those data are then combined with the prior distribution to form a *posterior distribution* for the same set of parameters, one which is hopefully more concentrated than the prior. Quantities calculated from this posterior distribution of the parameters form the basis of inference. Point estimates, for example, might be obtained by calculating the mean, median or mode of a parameter posterior distribution, while parameter precision might be estimated by the standard deviation or some suitable interquantile range.

From a Bayesian perspective, both observed data and parameters are considered as random quantities. This allows legitimate statements to be made about, say, the probability of a hypothesis being true, which is not, of course, so when using a frequentist approach. Formally, the transition from prior distribution to posterior distribution involves the following application of *Bayes' theorem*:

$$P(\theta \mid D) = \frac{P(\theta)P(D \mid \theta)}{\int P(\theta)P(D \mid \theta)d\theta} \tag{8.1}$$

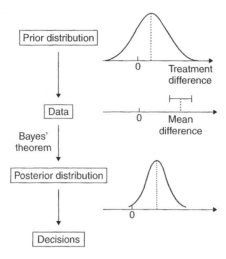

Figure 8.1   Conceptual framework for Bayesian analysis.

where $P(\theta|D)$ is the posterior distribution of the parameters θ given the data D, and $P(\theta)$ is the prior distribution of these parameters. The conditional probability $P(D|\theta)$ is what we generally term the *likelihood* of the data, so the rather technical looking (8.1) can be replaced by

$$posterior\ distribution \propto likelihood \times prior\ distribution \qquad (8.2)$$

The denominator in (8.1), the likelihood accumulated over all possible prior values, has been left out of (8.2) and the equality replaced by proportionality. The denominator is essentially a fixed normalizing factor which ensures that the posterior probabilities sum to one.

As an illustration of the mathematics of the Bayesian approach, we shall consider a sequence of *Bernoulli trials* – independent trials in which the result is either a 'success' or 'failure', with the same probability of success, θ, for all trials. We will assume that our prior knowledge about likely values of θ can be summarized in terms of a *beta distribution* for θ (this is suitable since a random variable having a beta distribution takes values between 0 and 1). Explicitly, the density function assumed for θ is then

$$P(\theta) = \frac{\theta^{\alpha-1}(1-\theta)^{\beta-1}\Gamma(\alpha+\beta)}{\Gamma(\alpha)\Gamma(\beta)} \qquad (8.3)$$

where Γ is the gamma function, and α and β are parameters which determine the form of $P(\theta)$. Figure 8.2 shows four beta densities. Symmetrical unimodal distributions are obtained for $\alpha = \beta > 1$, narrowing as their value increases; when $\alpha \neq \beta$ the distribution is asymmetrical. The mean and variance of a beta random variable are $\alpha/(\alpha + \beta)$ and $\alpha\beta/(\alpha + \beta)^2 (\alpha + \beta + 1)$, respectively.

If, in a sequence of n Bernoulli trials, we observe r successes, then the likelihood is proportional to $\theta^r(1 - \theta)^{n-r}$. Consequently the posterior distribution of θ is proportional to

$$\theta^{\alpha+r-1}(1-\theta)^{\beta+n-r+1} \qquad (8.4)$$

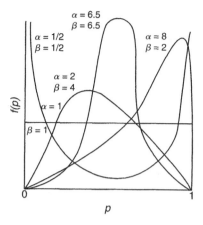

Figure 8.2 Four beta distributions.

which is another beta distribution with parameters $\alpha^* = \alpha + r$ and $\beta^* = \beta + n - r$. The mean of the posterior distribution is $(\alpha + r)/(\alpha + \beta + n)$; consequently, as α and β approach zero, corresponding to a prior distribution with the greatest possible variance, so the posterior mean approaches r/n, the estimate of θ that would be obtained by maximum likelihood. If one starts from a position of diffuse and uninformative prior distributions, then the focus of a Bayesian analysis is generally little different from that of other methods. As r and n increase relative to α and β, the variance of the posterior distribution approaches the familiar

$$\frac{r}{n}\left(1 - \frac{r}{n}\right)/n \qquad (8.5)$$

Figure 8.2 shows a beta distribution with $\alpha = \beta = 6.5$, the posterior distribution that would occur following the observation of 6 successes in 12 trials, with the use of the reasonably uninformative prior in which $\alpha = \beta = 0.5$ (also shown).

In this simple example involving Bernoulli trials, the posterior distribution takes a well-known form from which it was simple to extract the required mean, etc. In practice, however, this is not usually possible, and until relatively recently Bayesian statistics was little more than an intellectual curiosity, since the numerical integrations needed to deal with the posterior distribution meant that they could not be applied to real data sets. All this has now changed and recently developed computer-intensive sampling methods of estimation have revolutionized the application of Bayesian methods in statistics in general, and medical statistics in particular. The primary tools responsible for this revolution are *Markov chain Monte Carlo* (MCMC) methods. These methods are similar to Monte Carlo methods which estimate features of an unknown distribution by sampling from that distribution. For general distributions, however, Monte Carlo methods are difficult if not impossible to implement (e.g. for distributions of arbitrarily high dimension). MCMC methods overcome this limitation by constructing a suitable *Markov chain*, which is easy to sample from, and whose stationary distribution is the required posterior distribution, $P(\theta|D)$. The samples drawn from this constructed posterior distribution can then be used to estimate sample means, standard deviations and other qualities of interest about the parameters. For the theoretical background, see, for example, Roberts (1996).

One of the features of an MCMC procedure is that, regardless of where it is started, in the long run it tends to converge to the required stationary distribution. Thus the MCMC method consists of what is generally known as a 'burn-in' period during which it is hoped that the stationary distribution is reached, followed by a period of monitoring during which sample values of the quantities of interest are recorded and during which tests of convergence are undertaken. The latter is no formality when MCMC methods are being used, as some of the material in Gilks *et al.* (1996) demonstrates.

Several algorithms have been proposed for constructing Markov chains with speci-fied stationary distributions; these include the *Gibbs sampler* (Geman and Geman, 1984; Gelfand and Smith, 1990; Zeger and Karim, 1991), and *data augmentation methods* (Tanner and Wong, 1987). The Gibbs sampler leads to relatively straightfor-ward implementation even in situations which are intractable from other approaches because it reduces the problem to a simpler sequence of problems, each of which deals with one unknown quantity at a time.

One of the strengths of the MCMC approach is the ability to make inferences on arbitrary functions of unknown model parameters. As an example, consider a study involving three drug treatments A, B and C and a control treatment; a standard param-eterization would be a mean contrast for the effects of each drug relative to the com-mon control group. However, we might wish to know what the probability is that the pair of drugs that perform best in some small trial actually contains the 'best' drug. This kind of information is extremely valuable in drug development, but is not readily calculated from knowledge of the point estimates and covariance matrix of the stand-ard parameters. It is, however, an extremely simple task to monitor the *ranks* of the effects of each treatment from each MCMC sample, and to obtain an estimate of their distribution, confidence intervals and so on. An example of this approach is given later.

8.2.1   Examples of Bayesian estimation using Markov chain Monte Carlo

The example presented in this subsection is taken with permission from Spiegelhalter *et al.* (1996). The example involves mortality rates in 12 hospitals performing cardiac surgery in babies. The data are shown in Table 8.1. We shall consider both a fixed effects and random effects model for the data.

In the fixed effects model, the numbers of deaths r_i for hospital i are modelled as a binary response variable with true failure probability p_i. The latter are assumed to be

Table 8.1   Mortality rates in 12 hospitals performing cardiac surgery in babies

	Hospital											
	A	B	C	D	E	F	G	H	I	J	K	L
No. of operations (n)	47	148	119	810	211	196	148	215	207	97	256	360
No. of deaths (r)	0	18	8	46	8	13	9	31	14	8	29	24

independent for each hospital and to have a prior distribution which is a beta distribution with $\alpha = \beta = 1$.

Then we shall assume that failure rates across hospitals are similar in some way, and specify a random effects model for the true failure models, such that

$$\text{logit}(p_i) = b_i, \qquad b_i \sim N(\mu, \sigma) \qquad (8.6)$$

Here two parameters are involved, μ and σ, and both have to be assigned prior distributions. For μ a normal distribution with mean zero and large variance is used, and for σ a *gamma distribution*.

After a 500-iteration burn-in, a further 1000 iterations were used to provide the required posterior distributions for each model. Figure 8.3 shows the posterior mean 95% *credible interval* for the estimated surgical mortality rate in each hospital for both models. A credible region is essentially a Bayesian confidence interval, that is, an interval of the posterior distribution which specifies the range within which a parameter lies with a certain probability.

As mentioned previously, a particular strength of the MCMC approach is its ability to make inferences on arbitrary functions of unknown model parameters. We can illustrate this with the cardiac surgery data by computing the rank probability of failure for each hospital at each iteration. This yields a sample from the posterior distribution of the ranks which may be summarized to provide an estimate of the mean or median rank for each hospital, plus a 95% credible interval. The results are summarized in Figure 8.4, and reflect the typically large uncertainty associated with the rank position of each hospital.

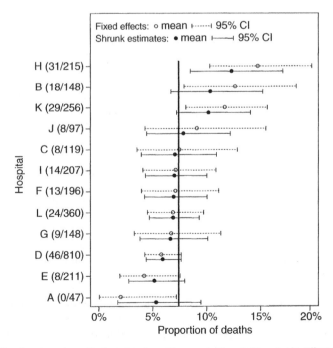

Figure 8.3   Fixed and random effects estimates of the surgical mortality rates in different hospitals. (*Source*: Spiegelhalter *et al.*, 1996, p. 17.)

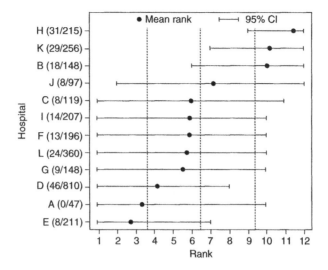

Figure 8.4   Posterior means and 95% credible regions for the rank of each hospital. (*Source*: Spiegelhalter *et al.*, 1996, p. 18.)

8.2.2   Informative priors

In the previous example the priors were essentially uninformative, chosen largely to keep parameters within a feasible space, and their presence within the analysis had very little influence on the eventual results. If, however, informative priors are to be considered, the statistician enters what is for many the rather unfamiliar territory relating to the characterization of prior beliefs. It is often convenient, both conceptually and in practice, to consider this process as one of translating prior beliefs into a hypothetical data set. This data set then informs a design in the same way that a meta-analysis of previous findings can inform a proposed study (see later in the chapter).

The choice of information source of a prior depends on the purpose to which it is to be put. For example, where studies are being undertaken within the context of an ongoing research programme, it makes sense to analyse and interpret the results of new studies as part of an ongoing accumulation of knowledge. However, while use of previous studies is appropriate in the assessment of final results, Freedman *et al.* (1994) suggest that such data should play a more minor role in monitoring a new study if it is to provide independent confirmation. (Freedman and Spiegelhalter, 1983, describe methods for eliciting subjective opinion. Stewart and Parmar, 1993, discuss issues in relation to using previous studies.)

To a Bayesian every problem is unique and is characterized by the investigator's beliefs about the parameters expressed in the prior distribution assumed in the specific investigation. The advantages of the Bayesian approach have been discussed above, but there are disadvantages, the most telling of which involve questions such as 'what will happen if your prior is wrong?' or 'if I were a medical control agency, to what extent would I trust your prior?' Certainly clinicians may express scepticism over the way different priors, purporting to represent belief, can influence the interpretation of results, and the results of a Bayesian analysis which has a chance of persuading sceptics and enthusiasts alike needs careful reporting. Freedman *et al.* (1994), for example, suggest that results sections should include the usual tables, plots, estimates and standard errors based on the data, and that interpretation sections should describe prior distributions and give treatment difference estimates (point and interval) using both an uninformative prior, and informative priors elicited perhaps from clinicians who favour one treatment over the other, and from those who do not. See Everitt and Pickles (2000) for a fuller discussion of these issues.

8.3 Meta-analysis

Everitt (1998) defines meta-analysis as follows:

> A collection of techniques whereby the results of two or more independent studies are statistically combined to yield an overall answer to a question of interest. The rationale behind this approach is to provide a test with more power than is provided by the separate studies themselves. The procedure has become increasingly popular in the last decade or so but it is not without its critics particularly because of the difficulties of knowing which studies should be included and to which population final results actually apply.

In essence, meta-analysis is a more systematic approach to combining evidence from multiple research projects than the classical review article. Chalmers and Lau (1993) make the point that both approaches can be biased, but that at least the writer of a meta-analytic paper is required by the rudimentary standards of the discipline to give the data on which the conclusions are based, and to defend the development of these conclusions by giving evidence that all available data are included, or to give the reasons for not including the data. In contrast, the typical reviewer arrives at conclusions that may be biased and then selects data to back them up. Chalmers and Lau conclude:

> It seems obvious that a discipline which requires that all available data be revealed and included in an analysis has an advantage over one that has traditionally not presented analyses of all the data on which conclusions are based.

Quantitative methods available for combining research findings from repeated studies have expanded in scope enormously over the last 15 years or so. The general feeling is that meta-analysis is likely to have an objectivity that is inevitably lacking in literature reviews and can also achieve greater precision and generalizability of findings than any single study. Consequently, it is not surprising that the technique has become one of the greatest growth areas in medical research. Examples of its use are available in Chalmers (1987), Der Simonian and Laird (1986), Sutton *et al.* (2000), and Sutton and Abrams (2001).

Meta-analysis has a number of aims:

- to review systematically the available evidence from a particular research area;
- to provide quantitative summaries of the results from each study;
- to combine the results across studies if appropriate – by combining results, more statistical power for deciding, for example, treatment effects is available and the precision of such effects is enhanced.

Examples of meta-analysis abound in medical research – particularly in systematic reviews of clinical trials and epidemiological studies. Meta-analysis of clinical trials, for example, has made an impact largely because so many trials are too small for adequate conclusions to be drawn about potentially small advantages of particular therapies. Advocacy of large trials is a natural response to the situation, but it is not always possible to launch very large trials before therapies become widely accepted or rejected prematurely. In fact, there are now several instances of very large trials being started after meta-analysis of multiple small ones was strongly positive (see Antman *et al.*, 1992).

Meta-analysis discourages the common simplistic and misleading interpretation that the results of individual clinical trials are in conflict because some are labelled 'positive' (that is statistically significant) and others 'negative' (that is statistically non-significant), but allows the investigation of sources of possible heterogeneity in the results from different trials.

Perhaps the most important aspect of a meta-analysis is study selection. Selection is a matter of inclusion and exclusion and the judgements required are, at times, problematic. But we shall say nothing about this fundamental component of a meta-analysis here since it has been comprehensively dealt with by a number of authors, including Chalmers and Lau (1993) and Petitti (2000). Instead we shall give a brief account of the statistics of meta-analysis and discuss a number of numerical examples, before considering a potentially fatal problem of the approach, namely *publication bias.*

8.3.1   Statistics of meta-analysis

Two models that are frequently used in the meta-analysis of medical studies are the *fixed effects* and *random effects* models. The former assumes that the true effect is the same for all studies, whereas the latter assumes that individual studies have different effect sizes that vary randomly around the overall mean effect size. Thus the random effects model specifically allows for the existence of *between-study heterogeneity* as well as *within-study variability*. DeMets (1987) and Bailey (1987) discuss the strengths and weaknesses of the two competing models. Bailey suggests that when the research question involves extrapolation to the future – whether the treatment *will* have an effect, on average – the random effects model for the studies is the appropriate one. The research question implicitly assumes that there is a population of studies from which those analysed in the meta-analysis were sampled, and anticipates future studies being conducted or previously unknown studies being uncovered.

When the research question concerns whether treatment *has* produced an effect, on average, *in the set of studies being analysed*, the fixed effects model for the studies may be the appropriate one; here there is no interest in generalizing the results to other studies.

Many statisticians believe, however, that random effects models are more appropriate than fixed effects models for meta-analysis because between-study variation is an important source of uncertainty that should not be ignored, in assigning uncertainty into pooled results (see, for example, Meir, 1987). A number of authors, for example Der Simonian and Laird (1986), have suggested conducting a test of homogeneity, that is, a test that the between-study variance component is zero, and using a fixed effects model if the variance component is not statistically significant. Such a test is described below, but, because of its likely low power to detect departures from homogeneity, its practical importance is probably limited.

The fixed effects model uses as its estimate of the common pooled effect, $\overline{Y}$, a weighted average of the individual study effects, the weights being inversely proportional to the within-study variances. Specifically,

$$\bar{Y} = \frac{\sum_{i=1}^{K} W_i Y_i}{\sum_{i=1}^{K} W_i} \tag{8.7}$$

where K is the number of the studies in the meta-analysis, Y_i is the effect size estimated in the ith study (this might be a log odds ratio, relative risk, or difference in means, for example), and $W = 1/V_i$ where V_i is the within-study estimate of variance of Y_i for the ith study. The estimated variance of $\bar{Y}$ is given by

$$\mathrm{Var}(\bar{Y}) = \frac{1}{\sum_{i=1}^{K} W_i} \tag{8.8}$$

From (8.7) and (8.8) a confidence interval for the pooled effect can be constructed in the usual way.

The random effects model has the form

$$Y_i = \mu_i + \sigma_i \varepsilon_i, \qquad \varepsilon_i \sim N(0,1),$$
$$\mu_i \sim N(\mu, \tau^2), \qquad i = 1, \dots, K \tag{8.9}$$

Unlike the fixed effects model, the effect size is not assumed constant across the individual studies. The true effects in each study, the μ_i, are assumed to have been sampled from a distribution of effects assumed to be normal with mean μ and variance τ^2. The estimate of μ is that given in (8.7), but in this case the weights are given by

$$W_i^* = \frac{1}{V_i + \hat{\tau}^2} \tag{8.10}$$

where $\hat{\tau}^2$ is an estimate of the between-study variance. Der Simonian and Laird (1986) derive a suitable estimator for $\hat{\tau}^2$:

$$\hat{\tau}^2 = \begin{cases} 0 & \text{if } Q \le K-1 \\ [Q-(K-1)]/U & \text{if } Q > K - 1 \end{cases} \tag{8.11}$$

where

$$Q = \sum_{i=1}^{K} W_i(Y_i - \bar{Y})^2 \tag{8.12}$$

and

$$U = (K-1)\left[\bar{W} - \frac{S_W^2}{K\bar{W}}\right] \tag{8.13}$$

with $\bar{W}$ and S_W^2 being the mean and variance of the weights W_i. An alternative estimator of τ^2 is described in Biggerstaff and Tweedie (1997). (Note that if $\hat{\tau} = 0$, then the random effects model is identical to the fixed effects model.) Allowing for this extra between-study variation has the effect of reducing the relative weighting given to the more precise studies. The random effects model produces a more conservative confidence interval for the pooled effect size.

A test for homogeneity of studies is provided by the statistic Q given in (8.12). The hypothesis of a common effect size is rejected if Q exceeds X^2_{K-1} at the chosen significance level.

A Bayesian dimension can be added to the random effects model by allowing the parameters of the model to have prior distributions. Some examples are given in Sutton and Abrams (2001).

8.3.2   Some examples of the application of meta-analysis

The data shown in Table 8.2 arise from a meta-analysis reported by Cottingham and Hunter (1992), concerned with the possible association between *Chlamydia trachomatis* and oral contraceptive use. The statistics are extracted from 28 case–control studies. A plot of the confidence intervals for the log odds ratio using the data from each study is shown in Figure 8.5. The impression is of a distinct positive association.

The results of applying both the fixed effects and random effects models described above to the data in Table 8.2 are shown in Table 8.3. The summary odds ratio calculated from each model is highly significant, giving clear evidence of a positive association between *Chlamydia trachomatis* and oral contraceptive use. The statistic for testing homogeneity takes the value 32.91 which, tested as a chi-square with 27 df, is not significant. There is no statistical evidence of heterogeneity.

As a further example of meta-analysis we shall use the results shown in Table 8.4, taken from studies addressing the possibility of an association between chlorination by-products in drinking water and colorectal cancer. The measure of effect size is again the log odds ratio. A plot of confidence intervals of this statistic for each study is shown in Figure 8.6. There appears to be some evidence of a positive association, although several of the confidence intervals are relatively wide.

The results of fitting the fixed and random effects model in this case are shown in Table 8.5. The test for heterogeneity is highly significant ($Q = 43.95$, $p < 0.001$), suggesting we should concentrate on the results from the random effects model; this

Table 8.2   Effect sizes and variances from 28 case–control studies of the association between *Chlamydia trachomatis* and oral contraceptive use

Log odds ratio	Variance	Log odds ratio	Variance
0.72	0.026	0.26	0.135
0.99	0.035	0.94	0.154
0.41	0.035	1.21	0.156
0.97	0.052	−0.02	0.158
0.58	0.053	0.41	0.162
0.63	0.059	1.32	0.172
0.17	0.065	1.25	0.185
0.93	0.080	0.75	0.270
0.41	0.083	0.15	0.284
0.73	0.095	1.39	0.397
0.92	0.099	1.36	0.410
0.72	0.104	1.20	0.426
1.05	0.106	1.52	0.570
1.05	0.126	1.80	0.672

Source: Cottingham and Hunter (1992).

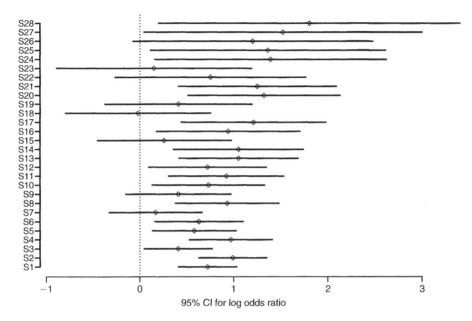

Figure 8.5 Plot of confidence intervals for the log odds ratios of the 28 case–control studies of *Chlamydia trachomatis* and oral contraceptive use.

Table 8.3 Results of fixed effects and random effects model applied to the data in Table 8.2

Study 1	Weights	
	Fixed effects (W)	Random effects (W*)
1	38.4615	21.2963
2	28.5214	17.8711
3	28.5714	17.8711
4	19.2308	13.7068
5	18.8679	13.5215
6	16.9492	12.5068
7	15.3846	11.6338
8	12.5000	9.9053
9	12.0482	9.6194
10	10.5263	8.5239
11	10.1010	8.3364
12	9.6154	8.0028
13	9.4340	7.8767
14	7.9365	6.8047
15	7.4074	6.4120
16	6.4935	5.7157
17	6.4103	5.6511
18	6.3291	5.5880
19	6.1728	5.4658
20	5.8140	5.1825
21	5.4054	4.8554

(*Continued*)

Table 8.3   (*Continued*)

Study 1	Weights	
	Fixed effects (W)	Random effects (W*)
22	3.7037	3.4369
23	3.5211	3.2792
24	2.5189	2.3926
25	2.4390	2.3204
26	2.3474	2.2374
27	1.7544	1.6822
28	1.4881	1.4431

Fixed effects estimates $\bar{Y} = 0.733$, $SE(\bar{Y}) = 0.058$, leading to a 95% CI for the odds ratio of (1.861, 2.333). Random effects estimates $\bar{Y} = 0.743$, $\hat{\tau}^2 = 0.021$, $SE(\bar{Y}) = 0.067$, leading to a 95% CI for the odds ratio of (1.845, 2.398).

Table 8.4   Results from 11 studies investigating the possible association between chlorination by-products in water and colorectal cancer

	Log odds ratio	Variance
1	−0.08	0.0015
2	0.12	0.0028
3	0.37	0.0076
4	0.54	0.0180
5	−0.03	0.0180
6	−0.11	0.0410
7	0.03	0.0460
8	0.34	0.1060
9	0.40	0.1000
10	0.30	0.0900
11	0.32	0.1500

suggests that there is some evidence for a positive association between chlorination by-products in drinking water and colorectal cancer.

The differences between the parameter estimates and standard errors provided by the two models in this example are highlighted by generating, from each model, bootstrap distributions for estimated effect size, estimated standard error and the ratio of effect size to standard error. The results are shown in Figure 8.7. The standard errors from the fixed effects model are more concentrated than those from the random effects model, and the resulting 'z statistics' from the fixed effects model much more widely spread.

Random effects models allow for heterogeneity between studies, but they do not offer any way of exploring and potentially explaining the reasons study results vary. Random effects models do not 'control for', 'adjust for' or 'explain away' heterogeneity, and understanding such heterogeneity should perhaps be seen as the main focus in many meta-analyses.

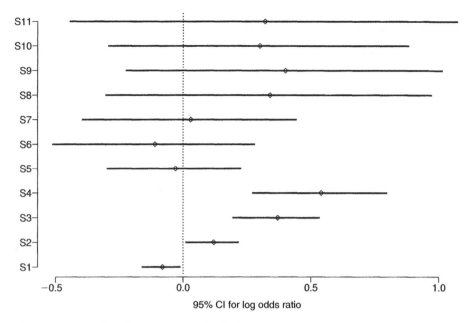

Figure 8.6 Plot of confidence intervals for the log odds ratios of the 11 studies of chlorination by-products in drinking water.

Table 8.5 Results of fixed effects and random effects models applied to data in Table 8.4

Study 1	Weights	
	Fixed effects (W)	Random effects (W^*)
1	666.67	25.71
2	357.14	24.88
3	131.58	22.22
4	55.56	18.05
5	55.56	18.05
6	24.39	12.76
7	21.74	11.99
8	9.43	6.97
9	10.00	7.28
10	11.11	7.85
11	6.67	5.34

Fixed effects estimates $\bar{Y} = 0.057$, $SE(\bar{Y}) = 0.027$, leading to a 95% CI for the odds ratio of (1.004, 1.116). Random effects estimates $\bar{Y} = 0.165$, $\hat{\tau}^2 = 0.037$, $SE(\bar{Y}) = 0.079$, leading to a 95% CI for the odds ratio of (1.010, 1.377).

The examination of heterogeneity only begins with formal statistical tests for its presence, and even in the absence of statistical evidence of heterogeneity, exploration of the relationship of effect size to study characteristics may still be valuable. There are many possible sources of heterogeneity: studies may differ in their design; studies

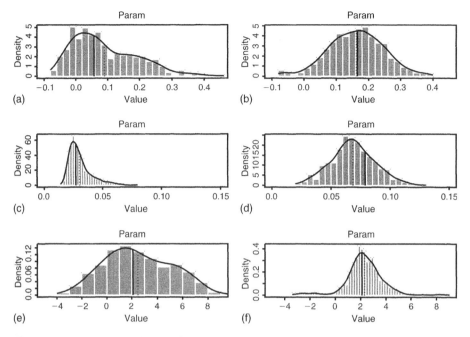

Figure 8.7 Bootstrap distributions for effect sizes, standard errors and *z* statistic for chlorination by-products and colorectal cancer data (1000 bootstrap samples used): (a) fixed effects, effect size; (b) random effects, effect size; (c) fixed effects, standard error; (d) random effects, standard error; (e) fixed effects, *z* statistic; (f) random effects, *z* statistic.

of the same type may differ in the success with which their study protocol was implemented; and studies may differ in the exact treatments involved. In addition, the effect of the intervention or risk factor may be different in different subgroups; if so, the results of studies with different proportions of people in the subgroups may differ in their estimates of effect size.

Examining how these various factors affect the estimated effect sizes in the studies chosen for a meta-analysis is of considerable importance, perhaps more important than the relatively simplistic use of meta-analysis to determine a single summary estimate of effect size. A range of examples are given in Petitti (2000); here we shall describe briefly a single example involving data from clinical trials of the efficacy of BCG vaccine in the treatment of tuberculosis, originally given in Colditz *et al.* (1994). The log odds ratios and associated standard errors from 13 studies are given in Table 8.6. In addition, this table contains the values of two covariates for each study, the geographic latitude of the place where the study was undertaken and the year of publication, which might be used to explain any heterogeneity among studies.

For these data the test statistic for heterogeneity takes the value 163.12 which, with 12 degrees of freedom, is highly significant; there is strong evidence of heterogeneity in the 13 studies. Applying the random effects model to the data gives the following results: an estimated effect size of -0.747, an estimated standard error of 0.192 and an estimated between-study variance 0.366.

To assess the effects of the two covariates on the effect sizes from each study, a weighted multiple linear regression was applied with weights given by

Table 8.6 Results from clinical trials on efficacy of BCG vaccine in the prevention of tuberculosis

Study	Log odds ratio	Standard error	Latitude	Year
1	−0.93869	0.5975952	44	48
2	−1.66619	0.4562127	55	49
3	−1.38629	0.6583388	42	60
4	−1.45644	0.1425132	52	77
5	−0.21914	0.2279254	13	73
6	−0.95812	0.0995490	44	53
7	−1.63378	0.4764557	19	73
8	0.01202	0.0633246	13	80
9	−0.47175	0.2387048	27	68
10	−1.40121	0.2746270	42	61
11	−0.34085	0.1119375	18	74
12	0.44663	0.7308625	33	69
13	−0.01734	0.2676565	33	76

Table 8.7 Results of weighted regression for effect size versus latitude and year for the data in Table 8.6

Term	Estimated regression coefficient	Standard error	Estimate/SE
Intercept	−0.469	1.602	−0.293
Latitude	−0.026	0.014	−1.887
Year	0.008	0.019	0.436

Multiple R-squared $= 0.439$.
F statistic 3.91 on 2 and 10 degrees of freedom, $p = 0.0557$.

$w_i = 1/(\hat{\sigma}^2 + s_i^2)$, $i = 1, \ldots, 13$, where $\hat{\sigma}^2$ is the estimated between-study variance and s_i^2 the estimated variance from the ith study. The results are given in Table 8.7. There is some evidence that latitude is associated with estimated effect size, the log odds ratio becoming increasingly negative as latitude increases (see Figure 8.8).

8.3.3 Selection of studies and publication bias

The selection of studies to be included in a meta-analysis will clearly have a bearing on the conclusions reached. Identifying studies through computerized bibliographic searches such as *Medline* is usually inadequate; it is often necessary to search reference lists and citations and to communicate with specialists in the area. But here we shall concentrate on possible publication bias in the studies selected, which is a major problem, perhaps *the* major problem in meta-analysis.

Ensuring that a meta-analysis is truly representative can be problematic. It has long been known that journal articles are not a representative sample of work addressed to any particular area of research (see, for example, Sterlin, 1959; Greenwald, 1975; Smith, 1980). Research with statistically significant results is potentially more likely to be submitted and published than work with null or non-significant results, particularly if the studies are small (Easterbrook *et al.*, 1991). The problem is made worse by the fact that many medical studies look at multiple outcomes, and there is a tendency

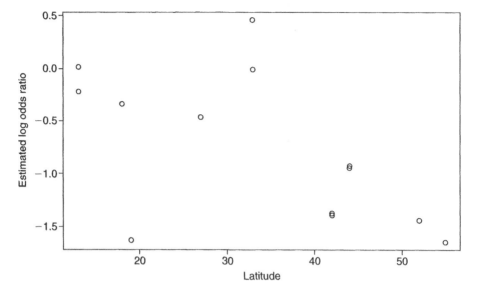

Figure 8.8 Plot of estimated log odds ratio against latitude for 13 studies of efficacy of BCG vaccine in the prevention of tuberculosis.

for only those suggesting a significant effect to be mentioned when the study is written up. Outcomes which show no clear treatment effect are often ignored, and so will not be included in any later review of studies looking at those particular outcomes. Publication bias is likely to lead to an over-representation of positive results.

Clearly, then, it becomes of some importance to assess the likelihood of publication bias in any meta-analysis. A well-known informal method of assessing publication bias is the so-called *funnel plot*, usually a plot of a measure of a study's precision, for example, one over the standard error, against effect size. The most precise estimates (for example those from the largest studies) will be at the top of the plot, and those from less precise or smaller studies at the bottom. The expectation of a 'funnel' shape in the plot relies on two empirical observations:

- The variances of studies in a meta-analysis are not identical, but are distributed in such a way that there are fewer precise studies and rather more imprecise studies.
- At any fixed level of variances, studies are symmetrically distributed around the true mean.

Evidence of publication bias is provided by an absence of studies on the left-hand side of the base of the funnel. The assumption is that, whether because of editorial policy or author inaction or other reasons, these studies (which are not statistically significant) are the ones that might not be published.

Figure 8.9 shows two funnel plots taken from Duval and Tweedie (2000). Figure 8.9(a) corresponds to the results from a simulation of 35 studies, and Figure 8.9(b) shows the corresponding plot with the 'leftmost' five studies suppressed. The data were generated to have zero effect size; the 95% confidence interval for all 35 studies using the random effects model was $(-0.018, 0.178)$; for the studies in Figure 8.9(b), using the same model, the corresponding confidence interval was $(0.037, 0.210)$.

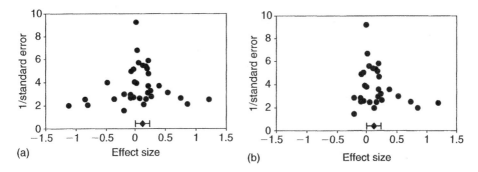

Figure 8.9   (a) Funnel plot of 35 simulated studies with a true effect size of zero; estimated effect size is 0.080 with a 95% confidence interval of $[-0.018, 0.178]$ (using the random effects model). (b) Funnel plot as in (a) with five 'leftmost' studies suppressed; overall effect size is now estimated as 0.124 with a 95% confidence interval of $[0.037, 0.210]$. (Taken with permission from Duval and Tweedie, 2000.)

Various suggestions have been made as to how to test for publication bias in a meta-analysis – see, for example, Begg (1994) and Egger *et al.* (1997). But the danger of the testing approach is the temptation to assume that, if the test is not significant, there is no problem, and consequently the possibility of publication bias can be ignored. In practice, publication bias is very likely to be endemic to all empirical research and so should be assumed present whatever the result of some testing procedure with low power.

So rather than simply testing for publication bias, several methods have been proposed for 'correcting' the problem. These include selection models using weighting functions (Hedges, 1984; Iyengar and Greenhouse, 1988; Dear and Begg, 1982; and Silliman, 1997a), Bayesian methods (Givens *et al.*, 1997; Silliman, 1997b) and the so-called 'trim-and-fill' methods (Taylor and Tweedie, 1998a, 1998b), but such methods necessarily make unverifiable assumptions and none will be discussed here. We will instead consider a more cautious approach suggested by Copas and Shi (2001), who propose a method whereby conclusions can be drawn from a meta-analysis under a variety of plausible possibilities for the extent of the publication bias, and then an assessment can be made of how different those conclusions are from one another and from the results of standard procedures.

The model proposed by Copas and Shi is based on the random effects model given in the previous section. This model is assumed to describe all the studies that have been carried out in the particular area of interest, but only some of these have been selected for review. To model the selection process a latent variable, z_i, is introduced; this is defined as follows:

$$z_i = a + \frac{b}{\sqrt{V_i}} + \delta_i, \qquad \delta_i \sim N(0,1), \mathrm{Corr}(\varepsilon_i, \delta_i) = \rho \qquad (8.14)$$

where the residuals ε_i from the random effects model in (8.9) and δ_i in the definition of z_i in (8.14) are assumed to be jointly normal. The role of (8.14) is that

$$Y_i \text{ is assumed observed only when } z_i > 0$$

The observed treatment effects are therefore modelled by the conditional distribution of Y_i given that z_i is positive. If $\rho = 0$ then this is the model without publication bias, Y_i and z_i are independent and so the outcome Y_i will have no effect on whether the paper is published or not. But when $\rho > 0$, selected studies will have $z > 0$ and so the corresponding value of δ, and consequently ε, is more likely to be positive, leading to a positive bias in Y. An explicit equation for this bias is given in Copas and Shi (2001).

The parameters a and b in (8.14) control the marginal probability that a study with within-study standard deviation V is published. Parameter a controls the overall proportion published, while b controls how the chance of publication depends on study size. With b positive, very large studies (very small V) are almost bound to be accepted for publication, but only a proportion of the smaller ones will be accepted. And if $\rho > 0$ then these smaller studies that are accepted will tend to be those with larger values of δ, hence larger values of ε and hence larger values of Y. Since we do not know how many unpublished studies there are, a and b cannot be estimated. But by considering the following equivalent way of writing (8.14),

$$\Pr(\text{select}|V) = \Pr(z > 0|V) = \Phi\left(a + \frac{b}{\sqrt{V}}\right) \qquad (8.15)$$

where Φ is the standard normal cumulative distribution function, we can select (a, b) pairs by setting suitable values for the selection probabilities. Operationally this is achieved by defining a series of selection probability pairs corresponding to what the investigator thinks is reasonable for the following:

$$\Pr(\text{select}|V = V_{\min}), \qquad \Pr(\text{select}|V = V_{\max}) \qquad (8.16)$$

where $V_{\min}$ and $V_{\max}$ are the minimum and maximum variances amongst the studies selected to be used in the meta-analysis. These can be converted into a range of values for a and b by solving (8.15); only pairs in which $b > 0$ are retained. (A numerical example is given in the next section.) For any given pair (a, b) maximum likelihood can be used to give estimates of μ, τ and ρ. Full details are given in Copas and Shi (2001).

8.3.4   Sensitivity analysis for publication bias

Figure 8.10 shows the funnel plot for the *Chlamydia trachomatis* meta-analysis studies. The plot gives little evidence of any substantial publication bias, but despite this we will still continue with the sensitivity analysis.

In this example we shall use five pairs of selection probabilities: $(0.99, 0.80)$, $(0.80, 0.50)$, $(0.60, 0.30)$, $(0.40, 0.10)$ and $(0.20, 0.01)$. These represent increasing degrees of publication bias. The minimum and maximum values of the variances of the 28 studies are 0.026 and 0.672. Consequently, for the first pair of selection probabilities, $(0.99, 0.80)$ we estimate a and b from the following two equations:

$$\Phi\left(a + \frac{b}{\sqrt{0.026}}\right) = 0.99$$

$$\Phi\left(a + \frac{b}{\sqrt{0.672}}\right) = 0.80 \qquad (8.17)$$

that is,

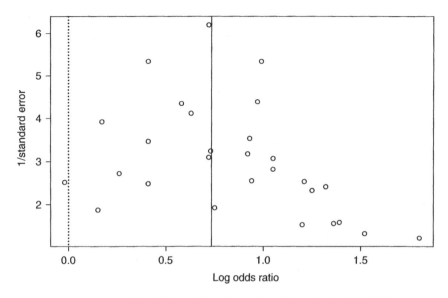

Figure 8.10   Funnel plot of the *Chlamydia trachomatis* studies, showing fixed effects estimate (solid line) and no effect (dotted line).

$$a + \frac{b}{\sqrt{0.026}} = 2.3263$$

$$a + \frac{b}{\sqrt{0.672}} = 0.84162 \tag{8.18}$$

leading to $a = 0.478$ and $b = 0.298$. The values of a and b calculated in this way for all pairs of selection probabilities are as follows:

Pair	Selection probabilities	a	b
1	(0.99, 0.80)	0.478	0.298
2	(0.80, 0.50)	−0.206	0.169
3	(0.60, 0.30)	−0.715	0.156
4	(0.40, 0.10)	−1.533	0.206
5	(0.20, 0.01)	−2.690	0.298

A sensitivity analysis now involves examining the dependence of $\hat{\mu}$ on a and b. The results of this analysis are given in Table 8.8. The last column in this table gives the estimated number of published and unpublished studies and is obtained from

$$\sum_{i=1}^{K} \{\Pr(\text{select} | V_i)\}^{-1} \tag{8.19}$$

(see Copas and Shi, 2001). We see from Table 8.8 that as the assumed publication bias becomes worse, the estimated effect size is considerably reduced, although the overall evidence of a positive association remains strong.

Table 8.8   Results of sensitivity analysis for publication bias on the *Chlamydia trachomatis* data

$\hat{\mu}$	p-value for $H_0: \mu = 0$	95% CI for $\hat{\mu}$	$\Pr(select \mid V_{min})$	$\Pr(select \mid V_{max})$	Estimated no of studies
0.741	<0.0001	(0.513, 0.951)	1.00	1.00	28
0.707	<0.0001	(0.497, 0.917)	0.99	0.80	31
0.617	<0.0001	(0.389, 0.844)	0.80	0.50	46
0.565	0.00015	(0.273, 0.856)	0.60	0.30	71
0.546	0.00055	(0.236, 0.856)	0.40	0.10	168
0.545	0.00064	(0.232, 0.858)	0.20	0.01	1055

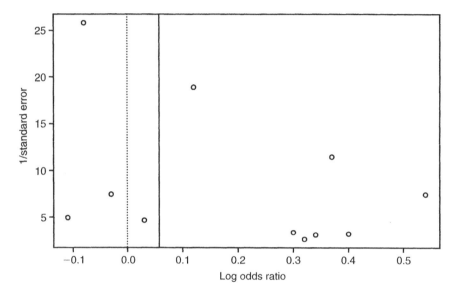

Figure 8.11   Funnel plot of the colorectal cancer studies, showing fixed effects estimate (solid line) and no effect (dotted line).

Table 8.9   Results of sensitivity analysis for chlorination by-products studies

$\hat{\mu}$	p-value for $H_0: \hat{\mu} = 0$	95% CI for $\hat{\mu}$	$\Pr(select \mid V_{min})$	$\Pr(select \mid V_{max})$	Estimated no of studies
0.163	0.039	(0.008, 0.318)	1.00	1.00	7
0.131	0.090	(−0.021, 0.283)	0.99	0.80	8
0.020	0.761	(−0.111, 0.152)	0.80	0.50	12
0.082	0.493	(−0.152, 0.316)	0.60	0.30	20
0.084	0.462	(−0.140, 0.308)	0.40	0.10	53
0.085	0.455	(−0.138, 0.307)	0.20	0.01	445

For the chlorination by-products data the funnel plot is shown in Figure 8.11. The number of studies here is relatively small, so the message to take from the funnel plot is not entirely clear – perhaps there is some evidence of publication bias. The results of the sensitivity analysis with the same values for the selection probabilities as used above, are shown in Table 8.9. Here the positive association estimated by the random effects model becomes non-significant if even the smallest amount of publication bias is present.

8.4 Summary

The Bayesian approach to the analysis of data from medical investigations is attractive in providing an integrated view, and is well suited to guiding the research strategy of a group of investigations sharing a common interest. Machin (1994), however, suggests that if the Bayesian approach is to evolve into more than an interesting but largely unused tool, there is a need for 'case' studies to illustrate what it gives above and beyond current methods. Certainly Bayesian methods have yet to gain wide acceptance in the public arena of, for example, clinical trials.

Meta-analysis has become one of the greatest growth areas in medical research, despite the many tough criticisms that have been levelled against it. An excellent recent account of the issues involved is given in Normand (1999). Various methods have been suggested for dealing with the thorny problem of publication bias, but the sensitivity analysis suggested by Copas and Shi (2001) appears to offer the most in practice by allowing investigators to examine how different amounts of publication bias affect their results.

Software

Specialized software packages are needed to fit the type of Bayesian models described in this chapter. Much meta-analysis can be carried out in a straightforward manner using a programming language as in the command line environment of S-PLUS, but specific meta-analysis packages are also available. Details are as follows:

BUGS   An interactive Windows program for Bayesian analysis of complex statistical models using Markov chain Monte Carlo techniques. An introduction and excellent sets of examples are available at http://www.mrc-bsu.cam.ac.uk/bugs/winbugs/contents.shtml.

Meta-analysis   A comprehensive meta-analysis package is available from Biostat, Inc., 14 North Dean Street, Englewood, NJ, 07631, USA.

S-PLUS   Code for the sensitivity analysis suggested by Copas and Shi (2001) is given at the end of their paper.

Exercises

8.1 Examine the effect of using different prior distribution for parameters in the Bayesian analysis of the mortality rates in Table 8.1.

8.2 The data below were collected for a meta-analysis of the effectiveness of aspirin (versus placebo) in preventing death after a myocardial infarction. Calculate the log(relative risk) for each study, and its variance, and then fit both a fixed effects and random effects model. Investigate the effect of possible publication bias using the approach described in the text.

			Survived	Died	Total
1	Elwood *et al.* (1974)	Aspirin	566	49	615
		Placebo	557	67	624
		Total	1 123	116	1 239
2	Coronary Drug Project Group (1976)	Aspirin	714	44	758
		Placebo	707	64	771
		Total	1 421	108	1 529
3	Elwood and Sweetman (1979)	Aspirin	730	102	832
		Placebo	724	126	850
		Total	1 454	228	1 682
4	Breddin *et al.* (1979)	Aspirin	285	32	317
		Placebo	271	38	309
		Total	556	70	626
5	Persantine-Aspirin Reinfarction Study	Aspirin	725	85	810
	Research Group (1980)	Placebo	354	52	406
		Total	1 079	137	1 216
6	Aspirin Myocardial Infarction	Aspirin	2 021	346	2 267
	Study Research Group (1980)	Placebo	2 038	219	2 257
		Total	4 059	465	4 524
7	ISIS-2 Collaborative Group (1988)	Aspirin	7 017	1 570	8 587
		Placebo	6 880	1 720	8 600
		Total	13 897	3 290	17 187

9

Exact Inference for Categorical Data

9.1 Introduction

A problem that arises in many medical investigations is how to deal with what we shall call *sparse data*. Such data can arise, of course, simply because the investigator collects only a small number of observations. But of more concern perhaps are situations where a rare event is being studied and large numbers of observations may only result in one or two events being recorded. For such data sets, methods that rely on deriving, say, *p*-values from the tail area of some limiting distribution under a large-sample assumption (*asymptotic p-values*), may give misleading results. That this is so has been known for some considerable time, as the following quotation from Fisher (1935) makes clear:

> The traditional machinery of statistical processes is wholly unsuited to the needs of practical research. Not only does it take a cannon to shoot a sparrow, but it misses the sparrow! The elaborate mechanism built on the theory of infinitely large samples is not accurate enough for simple laboratory data. Only by systematically tackling small problems on their merits does it seem possible to apply accurate tests to practical data.

Until recently the calculation of confidence intervals and *p*-values based on the true distribution of a test statistic (*exact p-values*) posed, in most situations, insurmountable computational problems and so asymptotic values had to be used in their place. For large and well-balanced data sets this is of no practical importance since the exact and asymptotic *p*-values are likely to be very similar. But for small, sparse, unbalanced data sets, the exact and asymptotic values may be quite different and might lead to different conclusions concerning the hypothesis of interest. Fortunately, as a result of the computational power of modern computers and the development of powerful algorithms implemented in easy-to-use software, it is now possible to calculate exact *p*-values (and corresponding confidence intervals) in many situations of interest, as we shall illustrate in this chapter.

9.2 Small expected values in contingency tables, Yates' correction and Fisher's exact test

Most readers will be familiar with the usual chi-square test for the independence of two categorical variables forming a two-dimensional contingency table. In the derivation

Table 9.1　Firefighters' entrance exam results

Test Results	Race				
	White	Black	Asian	Hispanic	Total
Pass	5	2	2	0	9
No show	0	1	0	1	2
Fail	0	2	3	4	9
Total	5	5	5	5	20

Table 9.2　Reference set of tables for data in Table 9.1

x_{11}	x_{12}	x_{13}	x_{14}	9
x_{21}	x_{22}	x_{23}	x_{24}	2
x_{31}	x_{32}	x_{33}	x_{34}	9
5	5	5	5	20

of the distribution of the appropriate test statistic, a continuous probability distribution, the chi-square, is used to approximate the true distribution of the test statistic. The p-value associated with the test statistic is then calculated under the assumption that there is a 'sufficiently large sample size'. Unfortunately, translating the latter phrase into something that is practically relevant has not been easy. One rule of thumb suggested by Cochran (1954) which has gained wide acceptance amongst medical researchers is that the minimum expected count for all cells should be at least 5. The problem with this rule is that it can be extremely conservative, and, in fact, Cochran gave a further rule of thumb that appears to have been largely ignored, namely that for tables larger than 2×2, a minimum expected count of 1 is permissible as long as no more than 20% of the cells have expected values below 5.

In the end no simple rule covers all cases, and it is difficult to identify, a priori, whether or not a given data set is likely to suffer from the usual asymptotic inference. This has led to suggestions for alternative test statistics which attempt to make the asymptotic p-value more accurate. The best known of these is *Yates' correction*. In addition, procedures not dependant on the latter, such as Fisher's exact test for 2×2 tables have been in use for many years.

Nowadays, however, an exact p-value can be calculated for *any* contingency table in which there is concern about the sparseness of the data. The main idea in evaluating the exact p-value is to evaluate the observed table relevant to a reference set of other tables of the same size that are like it in every possible respect, except in terms of the extent of departure from the null hypothesis. This approach can be made clearer if we use the specific (non-medical) example of the data in Table 9.1, which summarizes the results of an entrance exam for firefighters. The X^2 statistic for testing independence takes the value 11.56; the associated p-value is 0.073, leading to the conclusion that test result and ethnicity of candidate are independent. But here the number of cells in the table with expected values less than 5 is 12, that is all cells in the table.

The appropriate reference set of tables for this example consists of all tables of the form shown in Table 9.2 (all the counts represented in the table by the xs are, of course, assumed to be positive). The exact p-value is obtained by identifying all tables in the reference set whose X^2 values equal or exceed the value for the observed table,

Table 9.3   Two examples of tables in the reference set of data in Table 9.1

(a)				
5	2	2	0	9
0	0	0	2	2
0	3	3	3	9
5	5	5	5	20
(b)				
4	3	2	0	9
1	0	0	1	2
0	2	3	4	9
5	5	5	5	20

Table 9.4   Reference set for a hypothetical 6×6 contingency table

x_{11}	x_{12}	x_{13}	x_{14}	x_{15}	x_{16}	7
x_{21}	x_{22}	x_{23}	x_{24}	x_{25}	x_{26}	7
x_{31}	x_{32}	x_{33}	x_{34}	x_{35}	x_{36}	12
x_{41}	x_{42}	x_{43}	x_{44}	x_{45}	x_{46}	4
x_{51}	x_{52}	x_{53}	x_{54}	x_{55}	x_{56}	4
4	5	6	5	7	7	34

and summing the null probabilities of occurrence of these tables found from a *hypergeometric distribution* (see Glossary; and Everitt, 1998). For example, Table 9.3(a) is a member of the reference set and has a value of X^2 of 14.67. The exact probability of this table under the hypothesis of independence is 0.001 08, and because its X^2 value is more extreme than the value associated with the observed frequencies, it *will* contribute to the exact *p*-value. Again Table 9.3(b) is also a member of the reference set; but its X^2 value is 9.778 and so its null probability does *not* contribute to the exact *p*-value. The exact *p*-value calculated in this way is 0.0398, leading to the conclusion that test results and candidate ethnicity are not independent.

The problem in calculating exact *p*-values for contingency tables is entirely computational. For example, the number of tables in the reference set for Table 9.4 is 1.6 billion! In fact it was not until Mehta and Patel (1983) found a clever recursive method of summing the probabilities in the relevant tables that calculating exact *p*-values for contingency tables became feasible. But it is still not possible to use exact *p*-values for all cases when they are required; even the fastest algorithms available break down on some data sets. In such cases the exact *p*-value can be approximated, mostly very accurately, by the simple process of *sampling* from the reference set of all tables with the observed margins a large number of times; 10 000 is recommended. The result is what is termed a *Monte Carlo p-value*. Let us now move on to examine some examples of the use of exact *p*-values in practice.

9.3   Examples of the use of *p*-values

All the examples in this section are taken from Mehta and Patel (1996a) with the kind permission of the Cytel Software Corporation.

Table 9.5 Results from a clinical trial
with a binary response

Outcome	Drug A	Drug B
Improved	5	9
Not improved	6	1

Table 9.6 Left ventricular wall thickness versus sporting activity

Sports	Thickness (mm)		Total
	≥13	<13	
Weightlifting	1	6	7
Field wt. events	0	9	9
Wrestling/judo	0	16	16
Tae kwon do	1	16	17
Roller hockey	1	22	23
Team handball	1	25	26
Cross-country ski	1	30	31
Alpine skiing	0	32	32
Pentathlon	0	50	50
Roller skating	0	58	58
Equestrianism	0	28	28
Bobsledding	1	15	16
Volleyball	0	51	51
Diving	1	10	11
Boxing	0	14	14
Cycling	1	63	64
Water polo	0	21	21
Yachting	0	24	24
Canoeing	3	57	60
Fencing	1	41	42
Tennis	0	47	47
Rowing	4	91	95
Swimming	0	54	54
Soccer	0	62	62
Track	0	89	89

Source: Senchaudhuri *et al.* (1995).

We shall begin with the hypothetical data obtained from a clinical trial of two treat-ments with a binary endpoint, shown in Table 9.5. The X^2 statistic takes the value 4.677 with a single degree of freedom. The associated *p*-value is 0.0306, leading to the conclusion that improvement is associated with treatment and that drug B leads to a greater chance of improvement. The exact *p*-value, however, is 0.0635, suggesting that the evidence in favour of the superiority of drug B is far from convincing.

Our next example involves the data shown in Table 9.6. These data are given in Senchaudhuri *et al.* (1995) and report the thickness of the left ventricular wall, measured by echocardiography in 947 athletes participating in 25 different sports. There were 16 athletes with wall thickness 13 mm or greater, which is indicative of hypertrophic

Table 9.7 Results from a multi-centre trial

Test site	New drug		Control drug	
	Response	No	Response	No
1	0	15	0	15
2	0	39	6	32
3	1	20	3	18
4	1	14	2	15
5	1	20	2	19
6	0	12	2	10
7	3	49	10	42
8	0	19	2	17
9	1	14	0	15
10	2	26	2	27
11	0	19	2	18
12	0	12	1	11
13	0	24	5	19
14	2	10	2	11
15	0	14	11	3
16	0	53	4	48
17	0	20	0	20
18	0	21	0	21
19	1	50	1	48
20	0	13	1	13
21	0	13	1	13
22	0	21	0	21

cardiomyopathy. Interest lies in determining whether the presence of this condition is related to type of sport engaged in.

Here the X^2 statistic of the observed table is 33.52 with 24 df. The associated p-value is 0.094. A Monte Carlo estimate of the exact p-value based on sampling 10 000 tables from the reference set is 0.1079 with a 95% confidence interval of (0.0999, 0.1159). Here, despite the sparseness of the data the asymptotic and exact p-values are very close. Both lead to the conclusion that type of sport is independent of hypertrophic cardiomyopathy.

The final data set to be considered in this section is that shown in Table 9.7. These data give the distribution of favourable response to active and control treatments in a multi-centre randomized clinical trial. The data consist of twenty-two 2×2 contingency tables (one for each centre) relating treatment and response. Three questions are usually of interest concerning such stratified 2×2 tables:

- Is there any evidence of heterogeneity in the odds ratios associated with each table?
- If the odds ratios of the separate tables are homogeneous, is the common odds ratio different from one?
- If there is evidence that the common odds ratio differs from one, construct a suitable confidence interval for the statistic.

Breslow and Day (1980) describe a test for assessing the homogeneity of the odds ratio across strata. The exact form of the test statistic is rather complicated and so is not given here. Interested readers can find explicit formulae in Liu (1998). When data are sparse the Breslow–Day test is no longer strictly applicable, and a more appropriate test is that given by Zelen (1971).

For the data in Table 9.7 the Breslow–Day test gives an asymptotic p-value of 0.0785. This suggests that there is little evidence of heterogeneity in the odds ratios of the 22 sites. But the data are sparse and it would be wise to also look at the exact (Zelen) test. The Monte Carlo estimate and confidence interval for this exact value, based on 10 000 tables, are 0.0132 and (0.0126, 0.0138). This leads to rejection of the null hypothesis that the odds ratios in each site are equal. There is evidence of heterogeneity, and examination of the data suggests that it is site 15 that is the cause. For all the other sites there is a relatively low response rate for both the new and control drugs, but for site 15 the latter is 11/14 (79%).

Perhaps the data were recorded incorrectly and the value 11 should in fact be 1? Let us assume this was the case and amend the data accordingly. Now both tests of the homogeneity of the odds ratios give very similar p-values: the Breslow–Day asymptotic p-value is 0.3714, and the Zelen exact p-value 0.2995. There is no longer any evidence of heterogeneity in the odds ratios, and we might move on to produce an estimate and confidence interval for the assumed common odds ratio. As with p-values, confidence intervals can be asymptotic or exact. The exact confidence interval is obtained by using the reference sets for each table as described in Chapter 14 of Mehta and Patel (1996a). The asymptotic confidence interval is based on the well known *Mantel–Haenszel estimator* (see Breslow and Day, 1980). Here the values of both of these for the 'corrected' data set are very similar.

	Estimated odds ratio	95% CI
Exact	4.339	(2.219, 9.150)
Mantel–Haenszel	4.275	(2.236, 8.175)

9.4   Logistic regression and conditional logistic regression for sparse data

The examples used in this section are taken from Mehta and Patel (1996b) by kind permission of Cytel Software Corporation.

The data shown in Table 9.8 arise from a study in which investigators gathered data on 2493 patients, amongst whom 60 had an uncommon clinical illness known as

Table 9.8   Antibiotics and diarrhoea

Diarrhoea	Cephalexin	Clindomycin	Age	LOS
0/371	0	0	0	0
4/219	0	0	0	1
2/774	0	0	1	0
31/1011	0	0	1	1
0/14	0	1	0	0
1/15	0	1	1	0
16/70	0	1	1	1
5/5	1	0	1	1

Antibiotics:	1 = exposed, 0 = not exposed.
Age:	1 = over 50, 0 = below 50.
LOS (length of stay):	1 = more than one week, 0 = less than one week.
Source:	Mehta and Patel (1996a).

clostridium difficile colitis, an acute form of diarrhoea associated with long-term hospitalized patients exposed to antibiotics. (The data are taken from Mehta and Patel, 1996a). Interest lies in assessing the effects of age, length of hospital stay and exposure to clindamycin and cephalexin, two antibiotics, on diarrhoea. This is a relatively large data set, but few of the patients suffer from diarrhoea – only 2.4%.

The usual approach to analysis would be to apply logistic regression, estimating the regression coefficients of the four covariates by maximum likelihood. But this approach causes problems primarily due to exposure to the antibiotic cephalexin being a perfect predictor – all five patients exposed get diarrhoea. So what can be done? Again the solution is to use an exact approach via either *conditional likelihood* or what is known as *median unbiased estimation*; the details are, however, complex and so we simply refer readers to Hirji (1992) and Hirji *et al.* (1998). The results of applying this approach are given in Table 9.9.

These reveal that even after adjusting for the effects of age, LOS and clindamycin, exposure to cephalexin is of overwhelming importance. For patients exposed to this antibiotic the odds of suffering diarrhoea to being diarrhoea-free are at least 26 times the corresponding odds when not exposed.

Our next example involves data from a case–control study reported by Stanta and Walker (1986). The data consisted of 18 matched sets containing a total of 18 cases of lung cancer and 52 controls. The primary aim of the study was to assess the risk of developing lung cancer in women who had previously suffered from breast cancer. The covariates were radiation therapy for breast cancer and smoking history. Matching was based on age and date of diagnosis of the breast cancer. The data are given in Table 9.10.

Since the case–control sets have been matched on variables that are believed to be associated with disease status, the sets can be thought of as strata with individuals in one stratum having perhaps higher (or lower) odds of being a case than those in another after controlling for exposures. A suitable logistic regression model would need to include stratification parameters; the simplest model would be one with one parameter for the stratum-specific effect and constant slope across strata for the covariates, namely

$$\text{logit}[\Pr(y_{ik} = 1)] = \beta_0 + \alpha_k + \boldsymbol{\beta}'\mathbf{x}_{ik} \tag{9.1}$$

where y_{ik} is an indicator of 'caseness', taking the value 1 if individual i in matched set k is a case, α_k is the stratum parameter for matched set k, $\boldsymbol{\beta}$ is the vector of regression parameters for the explanatory variables, and $\mathbf{x}_{ik}$ contains the covariate values for the ith individual in matched set k. Such a model could be fitted in the usual way (ignoring for the moment the sparseness of the data), but there is a potential problem, namely the number of parameters to be estimated. With the introduction of the stratum-specific effect there are an extra $K - 1$ parameters in the model, where K is the number of strata.

Table 9.9 Results of exact logistic regression for diarrhoea and antibiotics data

Covariate	Estimated regression coefficient	95% CI
Age	0.872	$(-0.076, 2.065)$
Cephalexin	5.302	$(3.2848, \infty)$
Clindamycin	2.208	$(1.530, 2.858)$
LOS	2.479	$(1.331, 4.102)$

Table 9.10   Radiation and lung cancer

Stratum	Case indicator	Smoking and radiation history			
		None	Radiation alone	Smoking alone	Both
1	Case	1	0	0	0
	Control	0	3	0	0
2	Case	0	0	0	1
	Control	0	1	0	0
3	Case	0	1	0	0
	Control	1	2	0	0
4	Case	0	0	0	1
	Control	0	3	0	0
5	Case	1	0	0	0
	Control	0	3	0	0
6	Case	0	0	0	1
	Control	0	2	0	1
7	Case	0	1	0	0
	Control	0	3	0	0
8	Case	0	0	0	1
	Control	0	3	0	0
9	Case	0	1	0	0
	Control	1	2	0	0
10	Case	0	1	0	0
	Control	1	1	1	0
11	Case	0	0	1	0
	Control	1	1	1	0
12	Case	0	1	0	0
	Control	0	3	0	0
13	Case	0	0	1	0
	Control	3	0	0	0
14	Case	0	0	0	1
	Control	0	2	0	1
15	Case	0	0	0	1
	Control	1	2	0	0
16	Case	0	1	0	0
	Control	1	2	0	0
17	Case	0	0	0	1
	Control	0	2	0	1
18	Case	0	0	0	1
	Control	0	3	0	0

Source: Stanta and Walker (1986).

In our example, this would result in estimating 17 extra parameters, quite a lot but perhaps not too difficult. But imagine another study involving, say, 100 or 1000 matched sets. The optimal properties of maximum likelihood estimation apply when the sample size is large and the number of parameters remains fixed. In a stratified data set, however, as the number of strata increases, so does the number of parameters. It can be shown (see, for example, Breslow and Day, 1980), that as a result very large biases can be introduced into the estimated regression coefficients. So what can be done? The answer is to use a technique known as *conditional logistic regression*.

The underlying rationale behind conditional logistic regression is to regard the stratum-specific parameters as parameters whose values are neither of interest to us

Table 9.11 Conditional logistic regression results for the data in Table 9.10

Covariate	Estimated regression coefficient	95% CI
(a) Unconditional (stratification parameters not given)		
Radiation	0.249	(−2.003, 2.501)
Smoking	4.815	(1.994, 7.637)
(b) Conditional		
Radiation	0.178	(−1.786, 2.142)
Smoking	3.033	(0.949, 5.116)

Table 9.12 Exact conditional logistic regression results for the data in Table 9.10

Covariate	Estimated regression coefficient	95% CI
Radiation	0.177	(−1.949, 2.991)
Smoking	2.969	(0.984, 6.755)

nor essential for the inferences of interest in the study – so called *nuisance parameters*. Consequently, we do not need to estimate them, in which case we can create a conditional likelihood which will yield maximum likelihood estimates of the regression coefficients that are consistent and asymptotically normal. Details of how this is done are given in Hosmer and Lemeshow (1989).

The results of estimating a conditional logistic regression model for the data in Table 9.10 are shown in Table 9.11. Also given in the latter are the results of an unconditional regression analysis of the data. The estimated regression coefficients for the two covariates are larger in the unconditional analysis, but each analysis demonstrates that smoking has the greatest effect on the chance of developing lung cancer.

Here the sparseness of the data might throw into doubt the asymptotic results of Table 9.11; if so, it is possible to apply an exact form of conditional logistic regression (see Gail *et al.*, 1981, for details). The results of this analysis are shown in Table 9.12. In this case the exact results are very similar to the conditional results in Table 9.11.

The final example in this chapter will involve the data shown in Table 9.13. These data arise from a case–control study reported in Gared (1988) that was designed to determine the role of birth complications in schizophrenics. The sample consisted of seven families with several siblings per family. An individual within a family was classified as normal or schizophrenic. A 'birth-complications index' was assigned to each individual, ranging in value from 0 (uncomplicated birth) to 15 (severely complicated birth).

The results of a logistic regression in which family is regarded simply as a categorical variable having six degrees of freedom and represented by six dummy variables in the usual way are shown in Table 9.14. The regression coefficient for birth complications is estimated as 0.512, with standard error 0.233. The associated *p*-value is 0.028, suggesting that the birth-complications index is predictive of the probability of having a child diagnosed as schizophrenic.

Analysing the data using conditional logistic regression gives the results shown in Table 9.15. The asymptotic confidence interval for the birth-complications index

Table 9.13   Birth complications and schizophrenia

Family ID	Birth-complications index	Number of siblings		
		Normal	Schizophrenic	Total
1	15	0	1	1
1	7	1	0	1
1	6	1	0	1
1	5	1	0	1
1	3	2	0	2
1	2	3	0	3
1	0	1	0	1
2	2	0	1	1
2	0	1	0	1
3	9	0	1	1
3	2	1	0	1
3	1	1	0	1
4	2	0	1	1
4	0	4	0	4
5	6	1	0	1
5	3	0	1	1
5	0	0	1	1
6	3	1	0	1
6	0	2	1	3
7	6	0	1	1
7	2	1	0	1

Source: Gared (1988).

Table 9.14   Results from fitting a logistic regression model including family and birth complications index to data in Table 9.13

Covariate	Estimated regression coefficient	Standard error	Estimate/SE
Birth complications	0.512	0.233	2.197
Family 1	−4.112	2.747	−1.497
Family 2	1.535	2.278	0.674
Family 3	−1.052	2.416	−0.435
Family 4	0.406	2.120	0.192
Family 5	1.458	2.183	0.668
Family 6	0.465	2.123	0.219

Table 9.15   Conditional logistic regression results for the data in Table 9.13

Covariate	Estimated regression coefficient	95% CI
(a) Asymptotic		
Birth complications	0.325	(−0.004, 0.654)
(b) Exact		
Birth complications	0.325	(0.022, 0.7407)

regression parameter just includes the value zero. The exact confidence interval, however, excludes zero. The exact analysis again suggests that there is evidence of a positive association between the chance of schizophrenia and the birth-complications index. The estimated odds ratio for an increase of one unit in the index is 1.384 with a 95% confidence interval of (1.022, 2.097).

9.5 Summary

Sparse data occur frequently in medical investigation. The methods described in this chapter provide a powerful tool for dealing with such data by providing exact p-values, parameter estimates and confidence intervals, rather than values based on an asymptotic approximation. In many cases using the exact approach can lead to different conclusions from those based on asymptotic p-values.

Software

The most extensive and comprehensive software for exact inference is that marketed by Cytel Software Corporation, 675 Massachusetts Avenue, Cambridge, MA 02139, USA (http://www.cytel.com). The two packages are **StatXact** and **LogXact**; accompanying manuals are excellent. LogXact is reviewed in Hardin (2000).

Exercises

9.1 The data below show the number of cases of bronchitis by level of organic particulates in the air and by age. Test whether there is any evidence of heterogeneity in the odds ratios, and, if not, estimate the common odds ratio and its 95% confidence interval.

Age	Organic particulates	Bronchitis	
		Yes	No
15–24	High	2	38
	Low	0	21
23–39	High	1	18
	Low	1	12
40–60	High	2	35
	Low	1	25
60+	High	2	20
	Low	1	18

9.2 In a study of non-metastatic osteogenic sarcoma, the investigators were interested in determining which of sex, osteoid pathology (AOP), and lymphocytic infiltration (LYINF) were the best predictors of a three-year disease-free internal (DFI3). Investigate the data below using a suitable form of logistic regression.

DFI3	LYINF	SEX	AOP
1	0	0	0
1	0	0	0
1	0	0	0
1	0	1	0
1	0	1	0
1	0	1	1
1	0	1	1
1	1	0	0
1	1	0	0
1	1	0	0
1	1	0	1
1	1	0	1
1	1	1	1
1	1	1	1
1	1	1	1
1	1	1	1
0	1	0	1
0	1	1	0
0	1	1	0
0	1	1	1
0	1	1	1
0	1	1	1
0	1	1	1

10

Finite Mixture Models

10.1 Introduction

In 1893 Professor W.R. Weldon examined a histogram of measurements of the ratio of forehead to body length of 1000 crabs sampled from the Bay of Naples, and noticed that it deviated markedly from that of a normal curve. Weldon speculated that the asymmetry in the histogram of these data might be an indication that this population was evolving toward two new subspecies. Aware of his own limited mathematical training, Weldon took the problem to his colleague Karl Pearson. Pearson (1894) suggested that a mixture of two normal probability density functions with different means, μ_1 and μ_2, different variances, σ_1^2 and σ_2^2, and in proportions p_1 and p_2 might explain the observed skewness in the data – a probability density function of the form

$$f(x) = p_1 N(x; \mu_1, \sigma_1^2) + p_2 N(x; \mu_2, \sigma_2^2) \tag{10.1}$$

where $p_2 = 1 - p_1$, and $N(x; \mu, \sigma^2)$ represents a normal density function with mean μ and variance σ^2.

Pearson used the method of moments to fit the mixture distribution to Weldon's data, and his analysis did suggest that the two-subspecies idea was correct. To find estimates of the five parameters in (10.1), Pearson heroically solved a ninth-degree polynomial. A frequency polygon of the crabs data is shown in Figure 10.1, along with plots of a single normal density, the mixture density fitted by Pearson and that given by maximum likelihood (see later).

In the intervening hundred years or so since the publication of Pearson's classic paper, finite mixture distributions, of which (10.1) is a simple example, have continued to be seen as an extremely flexible approach to modelling a wide variety of random phenomena; it is, however, only in the past decade that their potential has been fully appreciated, with successful applications in astronomy, economics, engineering, marketing, genetics, and, of course, medicine.

10.2 Finite mixture distributions

Finite mixtures are a family of probability density functions with the following general form:

$$f(\mathbf{x}; \mathbf{p}, \boldsymbol{\theta}) = \sum_{i=1}^{c} p_i f_i(\mathbf{x}; \boldsymbol{\theta}_i) \tag{10.2}$$

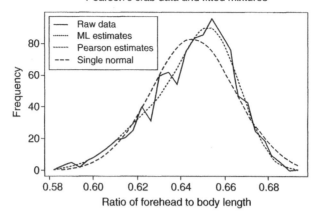

Figure 10.1 Frequency polygon of ratio of forehead to body length in 1000 crabs, fitted single normal density and two component mixtures fitted by moments and maximum likelihood.

where $\mathbf{x}$ is q-dimensional random variable, $\mathbf{p}' = [p_1, p_2, ..., p_{c-1}]$ and $\boldsymbol{\theta}' = [\boldsymbol{\theta}'_1, \boldsymbol{\theta}'_2, ..., \boldsymbol{\theta}'_c]$; the f_i are known as *component density functions*, and the p_i are such that $\sum_{i=1}^{c} p_i = 1$, where c is the number of components in the mixture. The general expression in (10.2) looks rather formidable, but if we compare it with the special case of the two-component, one-dimensional normal mixture in (10.1), where $q = 1$ and $c = 2, f_i$ is a normal density and $\boldsymbol{\theta}'_i = [\mu_i, \sigma_i]$, it becomes more transparent.

Finite mixture densities are most often used in one of the following situations:

- where the population in which the distribution of some variable or variables is to be modelled is known to consist of well-defined subpopulations, but the individual class memberships are unavailable. A simple example is a set of clinical measurements available for a number of patients known to have a variety of disease conditions, but where these conditions are unknown for the individual patients.
- where subpopulations are only suspected and finite mixture models are used to 'explore' the data for any potentially informative grouping. Here finite mixture densities act as models for *cluster analysis* (see Everitt *et al.*, 2001).

Mixtures in which the component densities are Gaussian (either univariate or multi-variate) are most commonly encountered in practice, as we shall see later, but mixtures with other forms for the component densities are now of increasing importance; again, examples will be described later.

10.3   Estimating the parameters in finite mixture models

Over the years a number of methods have been suggested for estimating the parameters in a finite mixture model. Pearson, for example, applied the method of moments, which leads to the need to find the roots of a ninth-degree polynomial to derive estimates for the five parameters in (10.1). Nowadays, the most common method of estimation is maximum likelihood using what is known as the *EM algorithm*. Full details of the process are available in McLachlan and Basford (1988) and McLachlan and

Peel (2000), but it is useful to give the basics of the method here. We shall consider a finite mixture model which consists of multivariate normal densities with mean vectors, $\boldsymbol{\mu}_i$, and covariance matrices, $\boldsymbol{\Sigma}_i$, as its components. For a sample of q-dimensional observations $\mathbf{x}_1, \mathbf{x}_2, ..., \mathbf{x}_n$ from the mixture, application of maximum likelihood leads to the following equations for estimation:

$$\hat{p}_j = \frac{1}{n}\sum_{i=1}^{n}\hat{\mathrm{Pr}}(j\,|\,\mathbf{x}_i)$$

$$\hat{\boldsymbol{\mu}}_j = \frac{1}{n\hat{p}_j}\sum_{i=1}^{n}\mathbf{x}_i\,\hat{\mathrm{Pr}}(j\,|\,\mathbf{x}_i) \tag{10.3}$$

$$\hat{\boldsymbol{\Sigma}}_j = \frac{1}{n\hat{p}_j}\sum_{i=1}^{n}(\mathbf{x}_i - \hat{\boldsymbol{\mu}}_j)(\mathbf{x}_i - \hat{\boldsymbol{\mu}}_j)'\hat{\mathrm{Pr}}(j\,|\,\mathbf{x}_i)$$

where $\hat{\mathrm{Pr}}(j\,|\,\mathbf{x}_i)$ is the estimated posterior probability of an observation $\mathbf{x}_i$ arising from component density j, and is given by

$$\hat{\mathrm{Pr}}(j\,|\,\mathbf{x}_i) = \frac{\hat{p}_j MVN(\mathbf{x}_i;\,\hat{\mathbf{m}}_j, \hat{\boldsymbol{\Sigma}}_j)}{\sum_{j=1}^{c}\hat{p}_j MVN(\mathbf{x}_i;\,\hat{\mathbf{m}}_j, \hat{\boldsymbol{\Sigma}}_j)} \tag{10.4}$$

where $MVN(\mathbf{x};\,\boldsymbol{\mu}, \boldsymbol{\Sigma})$ represents a multivariate normal density function with mean vector $\boldsymbol{\mu}$ and covariance matrix $\boldsymbol{\Sigma}$.

The equations given in (10.3) look ferocious, but they are, in fact, very similar to the likelihood estimation equations for the mean vector and covariance matrix of a single multivariate normal density, the only difference being the weighting by the estimated posterior probability.

Equations (10.3) do not, of course, give the required parameter estimates directly, since both right- and left-hand sides contain p_j, $\boldsymbol{\mu}_j$ and $\boldsymbol{\Sigma}_j$. The equations do, however, suggest the basis of an iterative scheme in which, given initial values of the unknown parameters, we can evaluate initial estimates of the posterior probabilities in (10.4), and these then can be inserted into the right-hand side of (10.3) to give revised estimates of p_j, $\boldsymbol{\mu}_j$ and $\boldsymbol{\Sigma}_j$. From these, new estimates of the posterior probabilities are derived and the procedure can be repeated until some suitable convergence criterion is satisfied. After convergence, a posterior probability can be calculated for each observation and each component density. These can be used to 'cluster' the observations by forming groups based on the maximum value amongst the estimated posterior probabilities of each observation.

In many applications of finite mixture models, a question that remains is how to estimate c, the number of components in the mixture. A likelihood ratio test is a natural candidate for testing, say, $c = c_0$ against $c = c_1 (c_1 > c_0)$, but this is well known to have problems in the context of finite mixture densities (see Everitt, 1996); nevertheless, the test can still often be useful as an informal indicator of number of components. One possibility for overcoming the potential difficulties with using the likelihood ratio test is to apply a bootstrap procedure; the value of the likelihood ratio is computed for each bootstrap sample after fitting mixture models for $c = c_0$ and $c = c_1$ in turn. The process is repeated independently a number of times to build up an empirically derived null distribution for the statistic. From this can be found an approximation to the p-value corresponding to the value of the likelihood ratio statistic of the original sample – see McLachlan (1987) and McLachlan and Peel (2000) for examples.

A variety of other ways for attempting to estimate the number of components in a mixture are described in McLachlan and Peel (2000). The problem is essentially equivalent to that of determining the number of clusters when using cluster analysis – see Everitt *et al.* (2001).

10.4　Some examples of the application of finite mixture densities in medical research

In this section we shall look at a variety of applications of finite mixture densities in medicine, beginning with one investigating the age of onset of schizophrenia.

10.4.1　Age of onset of schizophrenia

A sex difference in the age of onset of schizophrenia was noted by Kraepelin (1919). Subsequently, it has been one of the most consistent findings in the epidemiology of the disorder. Levine (1981) collated the results of seven studies on the age of onset of the illness, and 13 studies on age at first admission, and showed that all these studies were consistent in reporting an earlier onset of schizophrenia in men than in women. Levine suggested two competing models to explain these findings:

> The timing model states that schizophrenia is essentially the same disorder in the two sexes but has an early onset in men and a late onset in women … In contrast with the timing model, the subtype model posits two types of schizophrenia. One is characterised by early onset, typical symptoms, and poor premorbid competence, and the other by late onset, atypical symptoms, and good premorbid competence … the early onset, typical schizophrenia is largely a disorder of men, and late onset, atypical schizophrenia is largely a disorder in women.

The subtype model implies that the age of onset distribution for both male and female schizophrenics will be a mixture, with the mixing proportion for early onset schizophrenia being larger for men than for women. To investigate this model, ages of onset (determined as age on first admission) of 99 female and 152 male schizophrenics were fitted using a finite mixture distribution with normal components. The data are shown in Table 10.1, and the results of using maximum likelihood to estimate the parameters in the two-component normal mixture specified in (10.1) are given in Table 10.2. Confidence intervals were obtained by using the bootstrap (see Efron and Tibshirani, 1993). The bootstrap distributions for each parameter and data set are shown in Figures 10.2 and 10.3. Histograms of both data sets showing both the fitted two-component mixture distribution and a single normal fit are shown in Figure 10.4.

For both sets of data the likelihood ratio test provides strong evidence that a two-component mixture provides a better fit than a single normal. But it is difficult to draw convincing conclusions about the proposed subtype model of schizophrenia because of the very wide confidence intervals for the parameters. Far larger sample sizes than

Table 10.1 Age of onset of schizophrenia (years)

(a) Women

20	21	23	30	25	13	19	16	25	20	25	27	43	6	21	15	26	23	21	23	23
34	17	18	21	16	35	32	48	53	51	48	29	25	44	23	36	58	28	51	40	43
21	17	23	28	44	28	21	31	22	56	60	15	21	30	26	28	23	21	20	43	39
40	50	17	17	23	44	30	35	20	41	18	39	27	28	30	34	33	30	29	46	36
58	30	28	37	31	29	32	48	49	30											

(b) Men

21	23	21	27	24	20	12	15	19	21	22	19	24	9	19	18	17	23	17	23	19
37	22	24	19	22	19	16	16	18	16	33	22	23	10	14	15	20	11	25	9	22
25	20	22	23	24	29	24	22	26	20	25	17	25	28	22	22	23	35	16	29	33
15	29	29	24	39	10	20	23	15	18	20	21	30	21	18	19	15	19	18	25	17
15	27	18	43	20	17	21	5	27	25	18	24	33	32	29	34	20	21	31	22	15
27	23	47	17	21	16	21	19	31	34	23	23	20	21	18	26	30	17	21	19	22
52	24	19	19	33	32	29	58	39	42	32	32	46	38	44	35	45	41	31		

Table 10.2   Age of onset of schizophrenia: results of fitting finite mixture densities

Parameter	Initial value	Final value	Bootstrap 95% CI*
(a) Women			
p	0.5	0.74	(0.19, 0.83)
μ_1	25	24.80	(21.72, 27.51)
σ_1^2	10	42.75	(27.92, 85.31)
μ_2	50	46.45	(34.70, 50.50)
σ_2^2	10	49.90	(18.45, 132.40)
(b) Men			
p	0.5	0.51	(0.24, 0.77)
μ_1	25	20.25	(19.05, 22.06)
σ_1^2	10	9.42	(3.43, 36.70)
μ_2	50	27.76	(23.48, 34.67)
σ_2^2	10	112.24	(46.00, 176.39)

*Number of bootstrap samples used was 250.

those used here would be required to reach convincing conclusions about the competing models.

10.4.2   Variation of mortality rates between geographical areas

In this subsection we shall examine fitting mixture distributions to multivariate data concerned with the variation of mortality rates between geographical areas. Current residence is widely used for the comparison of incidence or mortality rates between geographical areas. When studying diseases with long latency periods, migration between geographical areas reduces the sensitivity of this method. Beginning in 1979, mortality statistics in the USA by state or country of birth were published by the US federal government and made available in computerized files. An analysis of residence histories provided in the US 1958 Current Population Survey found that 77.4% of people had not moved from their birthplace by the age of 19. Consequently, birthplace, which is listed on death certificates, provides a reasonably stable measure for geographical comparisons of potential early exposures for cohorts born before 1940, and Betemps and Buncher (1993) investigated state of birth as a possible risk factor for motor neurone disease (MND), Parkinson's disease (PD), multiple sclerosis (MS) and cerebrovascular disease (CVA). Using proportional mortality rates for each of the states in the USA except Hawaii, they found positive correlations between each disease rate and the latitudes and longitudes of the states, apart from CVA.

Here mixtures of multivariate normal densities will be used to 'explore' the structure of the four mortality rates for 48 states (Alaska and the District of Columbia are excluded). The relevant data are given in Table J of Betemps and Buncher's paper and are reproduced here in Table 10.3.

Two-, three- and four-component normal mixtures were fitted to the data with, in each case, the covariance matrices of the component densities constrained to be equal. With only 48 observations, allowing unequal covariance matrices would lead to far too many parameters to estimate. The parameters were estimated by maximum likelihood via the EM algorithm. (Equations (10.3) need to be amended somewhat to cope with the equal covariance constraint; details are given in Everitt and Hand, 1981.) For these

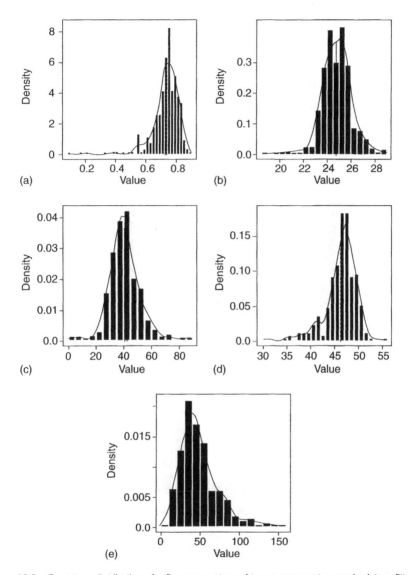

Figure 10.2 Bootstrap distributions for five parameters of two-component normal mixture fitted to the age of onset data for women: (a) mixing proportion; (b) mean of first distribution; (c) standard deviation of first distribution; (d) mean of second distribution; (e) standard deviation of second distribution.

data, the likelihood ratio test gives some weak evidence in favour of a two-component solution – see Table 10.4. The parameter estimates from fitting a two-component mixture are shown in Table 10.5.

The two-component solution corresponds to approximately equal division of the states into those with high CVA and low MS rates, and those where the reverse is the case. An obvious way to display the solution in this case is to identify the states belonging to each cluster (on the basis of the maximum values of the estimated posterior

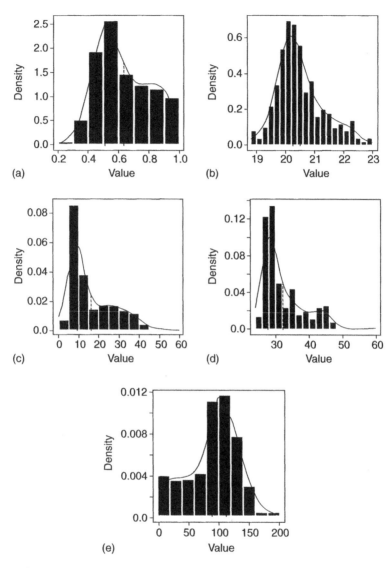

Figure 10.3   Bootstrap distributions for five parameters of two-component normal mixture fitted to the age of onset data for men (see Figure 10.2).

probabilities) on a map of the USA. This is done in Figure 10.5. There is a clear division of the states in terms of longitude and, in addition, amongst those states on the east coast, in terms of latitude. Florida differs from this overall pattern.

10.4.3   Using mixture distributions to model survival data

Mixture models can be used to analyse survival time data in a variety of situations. For example, Blackstone *et al.* (1986) consider that the risk of death following open-heart

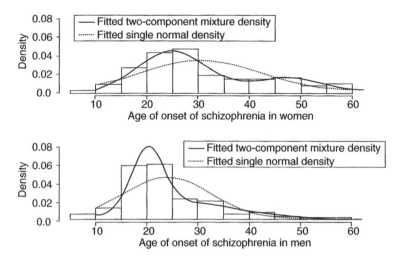

Figure 10.4 Histograms and fitted mixture distributions for age of onset data for women and men.

Table 10.3 Proportional mortality ratios per 10 000 from motor neurone disease (MND), Parkinson's disease (PD), multiple sclerosis (MS) and cerebrovascular disease (CVA) by US state of death

State of birth	MND	PD	MS	CVA
Alabama	12.15	20.29	5.41	942.54
Arizona	10.62	15.94	7.97	650.73
Arkansas	18.09	25.41	4.62	928.24
California	28.37	25.85	18.29	797.02
Colorado	10.98	31.11	20.13	755.86
Connecticut	19.55	24.88	11.26	753.64
Delaware	18.33	7.33	3.67	645.16
Florida	12.83	14.81	7.90	830.54
Georgia	12.95	18.01	4.42	1004.77
Idaho	26.80	37.11	16.49	828.87
Illinois	16.31	24.19	8.76	865.69
Indiana	12.35	29.05	9.61	974.09
Iowa	16.32	28.37	9.29	994.85
Kansas	19.32	32.32	9.48	955.63
Kentucky	17.14	18.72	3.83	915.26
Louisiana	15.95	18.76	1.41	910.33
Maine	16.46	22.86	8.23	787.38
Maryland	12.92	22.46	11.23	712.08
Massachusetts	19.33	22.31	10.20	721.93
Michigan	17.02	20.06	12.77	849.56
Minnesota	21.90	30.55	10.37	1011.33
Mississippi	13.20	23.10	3.85	964.53
Missouri	14.93	26.45	6.30	942.93
Montana	28.21	24.69	12.34	717.69
Nebraska	17.92	32.63	7.81	947.28
Nevada	12.09	12.09	12.09	677.15
New Hampshire	5.25	19.24	8.74	781.74

(Continued)

Table 10.3   *(Continued)*

State of birth	MND	PD	MS	CVA
New Jersey	18.16	19.76	11.75	731.49
New Mexico	21.67	32.51	14.45	680.87
New York	15.95	19.84	10.46	726.20
North Carolina	12.40	21.50	5.79	960.34
North Dakota	22.71	22.71	15.14	848.03
Ohio	19.24	21.48	11.60	868.26
Oklahoma	20.10	23.39	8.77	792.25
Oregon	23.67	29.89	11.21	833.33
Pennsylvania	14.44	21.65	8.39	780.15
Rhode Island	12.11	24.22	9.42	709.19
South Carolina	9.01	25.10	5.15	914.07
South Dakota	11.24	31.68	19.42	866.63
Tennessee	13.01	16.70	5.04	1007.91
Texas	16.31	23.63	5.20	933.55
Utah	16.70	44.95	12.84	909.32
Vermont	11.93	25.84	9.94	783.30
Virginia	17.35	23.13	3.40	925.51
Washington	24.34	21.09	12.97	800.68
West Virginia	12.56	16.37	6.85	781.56
Wisconsin	20.46	25.14	8.63	915.14
Wyoming	18.46	18.46	23.07	706.05

Source: Betemps and Buncher (1993, Table J).

Table 10.4   Results of likelihood ratio test for numbers of components in mortality data

No. of components	Log-likelihood	Chi-square	df	p
1	−537.62			
2	−529.80	13.84(1 v 2)	8	0.09
3	−522.16	13.37(3 v 2)	8	0.10
4	−518.65	6.07(4 v 3)	8	0.64

Table 10.5   Parameter estimates for two-component normal mixture fitted to mortality ratios data

Component	Mixing proportion	Means			
		MND	PD	MS	CVA
1	0.42	15.74	25.37	6.60	945.45
2	0.58	17.31	22.51	11.93	765.23
		Standard deviations			
		4.81	6.30	3.77	54.76

Correlation matrix:

$$\mathbf{R} = \begin{array}{c} \text{MND} \\ \text{PD} \\ \text{MS} \\ \text{CVA} \end{array} \begin{bmatrix} 1.00 & & & \\ 0.33 & 1.00 & & \\ 0.30 & 0.62 & 1.00 & \\ 0.10 & 0.24 & 0.17 & 1.00 \end{bmatrix}$$

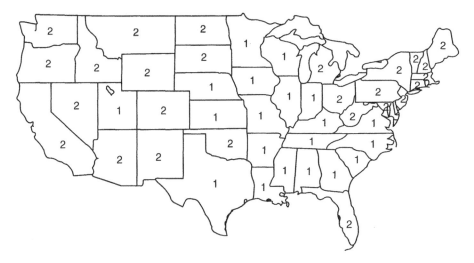

Figure 10.5   Two-component normal mixture clusters for the mortality ratios data, showing states assigned to each cluster on the basis of the maximum values of the estimated posterior probabilities.

surgery can be characterized by three merging phases: an early phase in which the risk is relatively high, a middle phase of constant risk, and finally a late phase in which the risk starts to increase as the patient ages. Here the use of a three-component mixture model with the components corresponding to the three risk phases can be an effective way of modelling survival – see, for example, McGiffin *et al.* (1993) and McLachlan and McGiffin (1994).

Mixture models for survival data are considered in detail in McLachlan and Peel (2000). We shall simply describe one example taken from McLachlan and McGiffin (1994), involving the distribution of the time to reoperation for degeneration of xenograft valves implanted in the aortic position of some 1004 patients. Of those patients who had their aortic valves replaced with xenograft prostheses, 73 underwent reoperations subsequently for xenograft degeneration, while 212 died without requiring a reoperation. The remaining 719 survival times were all censored in that, at the end of the study, they were either still living (without having undergone reoperation for xenograft degeneration) or had undergone a reoperation for some reason unrelated to xenograft degeneration.

For this problem, the failure time T is the time to the occurrence of the event reoperation for degeneration. Clearly, patients who die without a reoperation will never experience this event. Hence, in order to model the survivor function, $S(t)$, for this event, we can use a two-component mixture model of the form

$$S(t) = pS_1(t) + (1 - p)S_2(t) \tag{10.5}$$

where $S_1(t)$ is the survivor function for those patients who die without having undergone a reoperation for degeneration and $S_2(t)$ is the survivor function for the patients who undergo a reoperation in their lifetime; p is the probability that a patient will die without a reoperation for degeneration.

The survival time of those patients who never experience the event of interest is defined to be at infinity, and so $S_1(t)$ in (10.5) is set equal to one. The component $S_2(t)$ denotes the survivor function for time to reoperation for degeneration conditional on

Table 10.6   Results of fit of mixture model to xenograft prothesis data

Logistic parameters		Estimated time to reoperation		
β_0	β_1	γ	β_2	τ
−2.999	0.008	−0.004	−6.304	0.052
(0.663)	(0.001)	(0.001)	(0.502)	(0.005)

Source: McLachlan and McGiffin (1994).

the patient having undergone a reoperation in their lifetime. A suitable form for this component is the *Gompertz distribution* adjusted for the age of the patient at the time of the initial operation (see Gordon, 1990, for details); specifically, the form of $S_2(t)$ is

$$S_2(t) = \exp\left\{ \frac{-e^{\gamma x} e^\alpha (e^{\beta_2 t} - 1)}{\beta_2} \right\} \qquad (10.6)$$

where α, β_2 and γ are parameters to be estimated, and x denotes the age of the patient at the time of the initial operation. In this application, p is also modelled, as a logistic function of x:

$$p = \frac{\exp(\beta_0 + \beta_1 x)}{1 + \exp(\beta_0 + \beta_1 x)} \qquad (10.7)$$

The model can be fitted by maximum likelihood, with the results shown in Table 10.6; the standard errors shown were found by using the bootstrap, with 100 bootstrap samples. It can be seen that the age of the patient at the time of operation has a significant effect on the rate of degeneration of the xenograft replacement valve. And the estimate of the coefficient β_1 of age in the logistic model in (10.7) is positive (and significant), implying that the probability that a patient will need a reoperation for degeneration of the prosthesis decreases with age at operation. This is consistent with the fact that the older the patient is at the time of operation, the greater the chance that the patient will die before the xenograft prosthesis has degenerated sufficiently to necessitate a reoperation.

10.4.4   Using mixture models to identify regions of brain activation in functional magnetic resonance imaging

Functional magnetic resonance imaging (fMRI) is a non-invasive procedure for studying brain function; the technique gives images indicative of the relative proportions of blood oxy- and deoxyhaemoglobin, considered to relate to local neuronal function. There is an extensive literature on the many methods which have been proposed for using these images to identify brain regions 'activated' when a subject is performing a particular task; see, for example, Ford and Holmes (1998) and Rabe-Hesketh *et al.* (1998). We shall describe the use of a relatively straightforward finite mixture approach suggested by Everitt and Bullmore (1999).

In the experiment of interest, fMRI data were collected from a healthy male volunteer during a visual stimulation experiment (for details, see Everitt and Bullmore, 1999). A measure of the experimentally determined signal at each voxel in the image was calculated as described in Bullmore *et al.* (1996). Under the null hypothesis of no experimentally determined signal change (no activation), the derived statistic has a chi-square distribution with two degrees of freedom. Under the presence of an experimental effect (activation), however, the statistic has a non-central chi-square distribution (see Everitt, 1998). Consequently, it follows that the distribution of the statistic over all voxels in an image, both activated and non-activated, can be modelled by a mixture of those two component densities. So if p denotes the proportion of non-activated voxels in an image comprising n voxels in total, the mixture distribution assumed is

$$f(x; \lambda, p) = pf_1(x) + (1 - p)f_2(x; \lambda) \tag{10.8}$$

where f_1 is a chi-square distribution with two degrees of freedom and f_2 is a non-central chi-square distribution with non-centrality parameter λ. In essence, λ will be a measure of the experimental effect. Specifically,

$$f_1(x) = \frac{1}{2} e^{-x/2} \tag{10.9}$$

$$f_2(x) = \frac{1}{2} e^{-(x+\lambda)/2} \sum_{r=0}^{\infty} \frac{\lambda^r x^r}{2^{2r}(r!)^2} \tag{10.10}$$

Given the n observed values of the statistic, $x_1, x_2, \ldots, x_n$, the parameters p and λ can be estimated by maximizing the log-likelihood. Voxels can then be classified as activated or non-activated on the basis of the maximum values of the estimated posterior probabilities.

For the visual stimulation data this procedure led to estimates $\hat{p} = 0.96$ and $\hat{\lambda} = 3.467$. Voxels were classified as activated if their posterior probability of activation was greater than 0.5. Figure 10.6 shows the 'mixture model activation map' of the visual stimulation data for selected slices of the brain (activated voxels indicated).

10.5 Latent class analysis – mixtures for binary data

Multivariate data sets in which all the variables are binary are not uncommon in medical investigations. Mixture models with Gaussian components, for example, will not be suitable for such data. An alternative model which can be used is one in which the components of the mixture are *multivariate Bernoulli densities,* which take the form

$$\Pr(x_1, \ldots, x_q) = \prod_{j=1}^{q} \theta_j^{x_j} (1 - \theta_j)^{1-x_j} \tag{10.11}$$

The variables are assumed independent of one another and θ_j is the probability that the jth variable takes the value unity.

A mixture of such density functions is the basis of *latent class analysis* (Lazarfeld and Henry, 1968; Goodman, 1974), which assumes that the data consist of separate groups of observations within which the variables are independent – the so-called *conditional independence assumption.* Extending the nomenclature in (10.11) to accommodate the c components in the mixture, the assumed density function becomes

$$\Pr(x_1, \ldots, x_q) = \sum_{i=1}^{c} p_i \prod_{j=1}^{q} \theta_{ij}^{x_j} (1 - \theta_{ij})^{1-x_j} \tag{10.12}$$

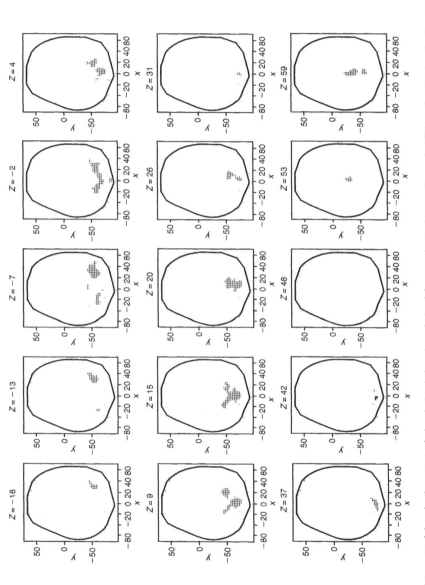

Figure 10.6 Mixture model activation map of visual simulation data derived from estimated posterior probabilities of activation for the 26 535 voxels. The threshold for posterior probabilities is 0.5. Each slice of data (Z) is displayed in the standard anatomical space of Talairach and Tournoux (1988).

Table 10.7   Response patterns for child and maternal reports of child and maternal smoking (1 = smoker, 0 = non-smoker)

x_1	x_2	x_3	x_4	Frequency
1	1	1	1	35
0	1	1	1	31
1	0	1	1	25
0	0	1	1	105
1	1	0	1	2
0	1	0	1	2
1	0	0	1	2
0	0	0	1	8
1	1	1	0	5
0	1	1	0	3
1	0	1	0	8
0	0	1	0	23
1	1	0	0	51
0	1	0	0	28
1	0	0	0	52
0	0	0	0	429

x_1 = child's report of child's smoking behaviour, x_2 = mother's report of child's smoking behaviour, x_3 = child's report of mother's smoking behaviour, x_4 = mother's report of mother's smoking behaviour. *Source*: Fergusson and Horwood (1989).

where, as usual, $\sum_{i=1}^{c} p_i = 1$, and now $\theta_{ij} = \Pr(x_j = 1 | \text{component } i)$. Estimation of the parameters in this mixture can be made using maximum likelihood in an analogous fashion to that described earlier for multivariate normal components.

To illustrate the use of latent class analysis we shall use some data reported in Fergusson and Horwood (1989); these data are shown in Table 10.7 and arise from mother and child reports of mother and child smoking behaviour. A latent class model with four classes was fitted to the data, in which the four classes (components) were assumed to be: mother smoker, child smoker (C1); mother non-smoker, child smoker (C2); mother smoker, child non-smoker (C3); mother non-smoker, child non-smoker (C4). It was further assumed that the reporting accuracies of child's report of child's smoking behaviour (x_1) and mother's report of child's smoking behaviour (x_2) do not depend on maternal smoking, and that the reporting accuracies of child's report of mother's smoking behaviour (x_3) and mother's report of mother's smoking behaviour (x_4) do not depend on child smoking. These assumptions imply the following constraints on the class probabilities:

$$P(x_1 = 1 | C1) = P(x_1 = 1 | C2)$$
$$P(x_2 = 1 | C1) = P(x_2 = 1 | C2)$$
$$P(x_1 = 1 | C3) = P(x_1 = 1 | C4)$$
$$P(x_2 = 1 | C3) = P(x_2 = 1 | C4)$$
$$P(x_3 = 1 | C1) = P(x_3 = 1 | C3) \tag{10.12}$$
$$P(x_4 = 1 | C1) = P(x_4 = 1 | C3)$$
$$P(x_3 = 1 | C2) = P(x_3 = 1 | C4)$$
$$P(x_4 = 1 | C2) = P(x_4 = 1 | C4)$$

Table 10.8   Estimated parameters for four-class model for smoking behaviour data

(1) Estimates of mixing proportions

Class 1 (C1)	Mother smoker, child smoker: $\hat{p}_1 = 0.147$
Class 2 (C2)	Mother non-smoker, child smoker: $\hat{p}_2 = 0.156$
Class 3 (C3)	Mother smoker, child non-smoker: $\hat{p}_3 = 0.140$
Class 4 (C4)	Mother non-smoker, child non-smoker: $\hat{p}_4 = 0.557$

(2) Estimates of class probabilities

Parameter	Value	Interpretation
$P(x_1 = 1\|C1) = P(x_1 = 1\|C2)$	0.593	True positive rate : child report of child
$P(x_2 = 1\|C1) = P(x_2 = 1\|C2)$	0.639	True positive rate : mother report of child
$P(x_1 = 1\|C3) = P(x_1 = 1\|C4)$	0.061	False positive rate : child report of child
$P(x_2 = 1\|C3) = P(x_2 = 1\|C4)$	0.000	False positive rate : mother report of child
$P(x_3 = 1\|C1) = P(x_3 = 1\|C3)$	0.950	True positive rate : child report of mother
$P(x_4 = 1\|C1) = P(x_4 = 1\|C3)$	0.888	True positive rate : mother report of mother
$P(x_3 = 1\|C2) = P(x_3 = 1\|C4)$	0.025	False positive rate : child report of mother
$P(x_4 = 1\|C2) = P(x_4 = 1\|C4)$	0.008	False positive rate : mother report of mother

where variable values of one indicate that the report identified the person involved as a smoker.

The estimated parameters in the model are shown in Table 10.8. The fitted model suggests that errors of measurements in reports of child smoking largely arise from false negative responses in which children who smoke describe themselves as non-smokers. Fergusson and Horwood show that one of the consequences of the high false negative rates is an underestimation of the prevalence of smoking behaviour and an underestimation of the strength of association between maternal and child smoking.

Other medical applications of latent class analysis are given in Pickering and Forbes (1984) and Formann and Kohlmann (1996).

10.6   Summary

The importance of finite mixture models in the analysis of particular types of medical data is reflected in the increasing number of examples to be found in the medical literature. This chapter has really only scratched the surface of the topic, and readers are referred to the excellent book by McLachlan and Peel (2000) for further details of important topics such as mixtures-of-experts models and Bayesian estimation, not covered in this chapter.

Software

Estimation of the parameters in finite mixture models does not seem to be available in any of the major packages; but there is a variety of software available for the fitting of mixtures models. Examples include the following.

NORMIX was the first program for clustering data that consist of mixtures of multivariate normal distributions. The program was originally written by John H. Wolfe in the 1960s (see Wolfe, 1970). A version that runs under MSDOS–Windows is available as freeware at http://alumni.caltech.edu/~wolfe/normix.htm.

Geoff McLachlan and colleagues have developed the EMMIX algorithm for the automatic fitting and testing of normal or *t*-component mixture models to multivariate data – see the algorithm description by McLachlan *et al.* (1998) at http://www.maths.uq.edu.au/~gjm/. The software plus user's guide (Peel and McLachlan, 1999) is freely available for non-commercial use on Geoff McLachlan's webpage.

Multimix is a Fortran program for maximum likelihood fitting of a class of models that includes latent class models and finite mixtures of multivariate normal distributions. The program was developed by Jorgensen and Hunt (1999) and the source code is available from Murray Jorgensen's website (http://www.stats.waikato.ac.nz/Staff/maj.html).

GLIMMIX is a program that implements the EM algorithm for the estimation of finite mixtures and mixtures of generalized linear models. The program allows for the specification of a number of distributions in the exponential family, including the normal, gamma, binomial, Poisson and multinomial. A demonstration version of the program can be obtained from http://www.gamma.rug.nl. The software is reviewed in Wedel (2001).

Mplus is a statistical modelling program which has its origin in structural equation modelling and was developed by Bengt and Linda Muthén (http://www.statmodel.com/mplus/index.html). Its modelling facilities contain latent class analysis. The facilities of the package are described in Muthén and Muthén (1998).

Exercises

10.1 Show how equations (10.3) have to be amended if the covariance matrices of the c component multivariate normal densities are assumed to be equal.

10.2 Use the bootstrap approach to investigate the distribution of the likelihood ratio test of two components versus one component for the age of onset data.

10.3 Fit two-, and three-component normal mixtures to the age of onset data, constraining the variables of each component to be the same. Use bootstrapping to find standard errors of the estimated parameters.

Glossary

Autoregressive process: A series of observations made in time in which the observation x_t at time t is postulated to be a linear function of previous values of the series; for example,

$$x_t = \beta x_{t-1} + \varepsilon_t$$

is a first-order or AR1 process.

Bayesian inference: An approach to inference based largely on Bayes' theorem and consisting of the following principal steps:

1. Obtain the likelihood, $f(\mathbf{x}|\boldsymbol{\theta})$, describing the process giving rise to the data $\mathbf{x}$ in terms of the unknown parameters $\boldsymbol{\theta}$.
2. Obtain the prior distribution, $f(\boldsymbol{\theta})$, expressing what is known about $\boldsymbol{\theta}$, prior to observing the data.
3. Apply Bayes' theorem to derive the posterior distribution, $f(\boldsymbol{\theta}|\mathbf{x})$, expressing what is known about $\boldsymbol{\theta}$ after observing the data.
4. Derive appropriate inference statements from the posterior distribution. These may include specific inferences such as point estimates, interval estimates or probabilities of hypotheses. If interest centres on particular components of $\boldsymbol{\theta}$ their posterior distribution is formed by integrating out the other parameters.

This form of inference differs from the classical form of frequentist inference in several respects, particularly the use of the prior distribution which is absent from the classical inference. It represents the investigator's knowledge about the parameters before seeing the data. Classical statistics uses only the likelihood. Consequently, to a Bayesian every problem is unique and is characterized by the investigator's beliefs about the parameters expressed in the prior distribution for the specific investigation.

Bernoulli trials: A series of n independent binary variables in which the jth observation can be labelled either 'success' or 'failure', and where the probability of a success, p, is the same for all trials.

Beta distribution: The probability distribution

$$f(x) = \frac{x^{\alpha-1}(1-x)^{\beta-1}}{B(\alpha,\beta)}, \qquad 0 \le x \le \alpha > 0, \beta > 0$$

where B is the beta function.

Binomial distribution: The distribution of the number of 'successes', X, in a series of n independent Bernoulli trials where the probability of success at each trial is p and the probability of failure is $q = 1 - p$. Specifically given by

$$\Pr(X = x) = \frac{n!}{x!(n-x)!} p^x q^{n-x}, \quad x = 0, 1, \ldots, n$$

The distribution has mean np and variance npq.

Exponential distribution: The probability distribution $f(x)$ given by

$$f(x) = \lambda e^{-\lambda x}, \quad x > 0$$

The mean of the distribution is $1/\lambda$ and its variance $1/\lambda^2$.

Exponential family: A family of probability distributions of the form

$$f(x) = \exp\{a(\theta)b(x) + c(\theta) + d(x)\}$$

where θ is a parameter and a, b, c and d known functions. The normal distribution, gamma distribution, binomial distribution and Poisson distribution are included as special cases. The binomial distribution, for example, can be written in this form as

$$\binom{n}{x} p^x (1-p)^{n-x} = \binom{n}{x} \exp\left\{ x \ln \frac{p}{1-p} + n \ln(1-p) \right\}$$

Fisher's exact test: An alternative procedure to use of the chi-square statistic for assessing the independence of two variables forming a 2×2 contingency table, particularly when the expected frequencies are small. The method consists of evaluating the sum of the probabilities associated with the observed table and all possible 2×2 tables that have the same row and column totals as the observed data but exhibit more extreme departure from independence. The probability of each table is calculated from the hypergeometric distribution.

Gamma distribution: The probability distribution

$$f(x) = \left(\frac{x}{\beta} \right)^{\gamma - 1} \frac{\exp(-x/\beta)}{\beta \Gamma(\gamma)}, \quad 0 \le x < \infty, \ \beta > 0, \ \gamma > 0$$

where Γ is the gamma function.

Hypergeometric distribution: A probability distribution associated with sampling without replacement from a population of finite size. If the population consists of r elements of one kind and $N - r$ of another, then the probability of finding x elements of the first kind when a random sample of size n is drawn is given by

$$P(x) = \frac{\binom{r}{x} \binom{N-r}{n-x}}{\binom{N}{n}}$$

The mean of x is nr/N and its variance is

$$\frac{nr}{N}\left(1 - \frac{r}{n}\right)\left(\frac{N-n}{N-1}\right)$$

When N is large and n is small compared to N, the hypergeometric distribution can be approximated by the binomial distribution.

Likelihood: The probability of a set of observations given the value of a set of parameters. For example, the likelihood of a random sample of n observations $x_1, x_2, ..., x_n$ from a probability density function $f(x;\theta)$ is given by

$$L = \prod_{i=1}^{n} f(x_i; \theta)$$

The likelihood forms the basis of maximum likelihood estimation.

Likelihood ratio test: A test of two competing models (M_1 and M_2) for a data set based on the ratio of the likelihood of the data under each model. The statistic

$$\lambda = -2\ln\frac{L_{M_1}}{L_{M_2}}$$

has approximately a chi-square distribution with degrees of freedom equal to the difference in the number of parameters in the two models.

Logistic transformation: A transformation, λ, of a proportion or probability, p, defined as

$$\lambda = \log\frac{p}{1-p}$$

As p varies between 0 and 1, λ varies between $-\infty$ and ∞. Plotting λ against p gives a sigmoid curve that is symmetric about $p = 0.5$. The reverse transformation is

$$p = \frac{\exp(\lambda)}{1 + \exp(\lambda)}$$

The logistic transformation is the basis of logistic regression.

Logrank test: A test for comparing two or more sets of survival times, to assess the null hypothesis that there is no difference in the survival experience of the individuals in the different groups.

Longitudinal studies: Studies in which measurements of the same variable at different time points are taken for each subject. Special statistical methods are often needed for the analysis of this type of data because the set of measurements on a subject will tend to be related (correlated) rather than independent. This correlation must be taken into account for valid scientific inferences to be made.

Mantel–Haenzel estimator: An estimator of the assumed common odds ratio in a series of 2×2 contingency tables arising from different populations – occupation, country of origin, etc. Specifically, the estimator is defined as

$$\omega = \sum_{i=1}^{k} a_i d_i \Big/ \sum_{i=1}^{k} c_i b_i$$

where k is the number of 2×2 tables involved and a_i, b_i, c_i, d_i are the four counts in the ith table.

Markov chain: A stochastic process such that the conditional probability distribution P of the chain at any future instance, given the present state, is unaffected by any additional knowledge of the past history of the system.

Maximum likelihood estimation: An estimation procedure involving maximization of the likelihood or log-likelihood with respect to the parameters involved. Such estimators are particularly important because of the many desirable statistical properties they possess. As an example, consider n observations from an exponential distribution of the form $\lambda e^{-\lambda x}$. The likelihood is

$$L = \prod_{i=1}^{n} \lambda x_i e^{-\lambda x_i}$$

The log-likelihood is

$$l = \sum_{i=1}^{n} \{\log \lambda + \log x_i - \lambda x_i\}$$

$$= n \log \lambda + \sum_{i=1}^{n} \log x_i - \lambda \sum x_i$$

Differentiating l with respect to λ leads to

$$\frac{\partial l}{\partial \lambda} = \frac{n}{\lambda} - \sum x_i$$

Setting $\partial l / \partial \lambda$ equal to zero leads to the estimator

$$\hat{\lambda} = \frac{n}{\sum x_i} = 1/\bar{x}$$

where $\bar{x}$ is the arithmetic mean of the n observations.

Median unbiased estimation: An estimation procedure in which the estimator, $\hat{\beta}$, of a parameter, β, is such that

$$\Pr(\hat{\beta} \le \beta) \ge \frac{1}{2}, \quad \Pr(\hat{\beta} \ge \beta) \ge \frac{1}{2}$$

Negative binomial distribution: The probability distribution of the number of failures, X, before the kth success in a sequence of Bernoulli trials where the probability of success on each trial is p and the probability of failure is $q = 1 - p$. The distribution is given by

$$Pr(X = x) = \binom{k + x - 1}{x - 1} p^k q^x, \quad 0 \leq x < \infty$$

The mean of the distribution is kq/p and its variance is kq/p^2. It is often used to model overdispersion in count data.

Nuisance parameter: A parameter of a model in which there is little or no scientific interest but whose values are usually needed (but in general are unknown) to make inferences about those parameters which are of interest. For example, the aim may be to draw an inference about the mean of a normal distribution when nothing certain is known about the variance. The likelihood for the mean, however, involves the variance, different values of which will lead to different likelihoods. To overcome the problem a search is made for test statistics, or estimations of the parameters that are of concern, which do not depend on the unwanted parameter(s).

Odds: The ratio of the probability of occurrence of an event to that of non-occurrence.

Odds ratio: The ratio of two odds, for example odds of an event for males and odds of the same event for females.

Partial likelihood: An approximate likelihood based on conditional probabilities, which is often used to eliminate nuisance parameters from consideration.

Poisson process: A process concerned with the random occurrence of events at points in time (or space), in which the number of events in time t has a Poisson distribution with mean λt, where λ is the constant intensity.

Posterior distributions: Probability distributions that summarize information about a random variable or parameter after having obtained new information from empirical data. Such distributions are used almost entirely within the context of Bayesian inference.

Probability sample: A sample obtained by a method in which every individual in a finite population has a known (but not necessarily equal) chance of being included in the sample.

Prior distributions: Probability distributions that summarize information about a random variable or parameter known or assumed, prior to obtaining information from empirical observations. Such distributions are used within the context of Bayesian inference.

Quasi-likelihood: A function, Q, that can be used in place of a conventional log-likelihood when it is not possible to make distributional assumptions about the observations, with the consequence that there is insufficient information to construct the likelihood proper. The function depends on assuming some relationship between the means and variances of the random variables involved.

Regression diagnostics: Procedures designed to investigate the assumptions underlying particular forms of regression analysis (e.g. homogeneity of variance or normality) or to examine the influence of particular data points or small groups of data points on the estimated regression coefficients.

Relative risk: A measure of the association between exposure to a particular factor and risk of a certain outcome, calculated as

$$\text{relative risk} = \frac{\text{incidence rate among exposed}}{\text{incidence rate among non-exposed}}$$

Thus a relative risk of 5, for example, means that an exposed person is 5 times as likely to have the disease than one who is not exposed. Relative risk does *not* measure the probability that someone with the factor will develop the disease. The disease may be rare among both the non-exposed and the exposed.

Residual: The difference between the observed value of a response variable (y_i) and the value predicted by some model of interest ($\hat{y}_i$). Examination of a set of residuals, usually by informal graphical techniques, allows the assumptions made in the model fitting exercise (e.g. homogeneity of variance or normality) to be checked.

Weighted regression: A form of regression in which estimates arise from minimizing a weighted sum of squares of differences between the response variable and its predicted value from the model under investigation. It is often used when the variance of the response variable is thought to change over the range of values of the explanatory variables, in which case the weights are generally taken to be the reciprocals of the variances.

Yates' correction: When testing for independence in a contingency table, a continuous probability distribution, namely the chi-square distribution, is used as an approximation to the discrete probability of observed frequencies, namely the multinomial distribution. To improve this approximation, Yates suggested a correction that involves subtracting 0.5 from the positive discrepancies (observed − expected) and adding 0.5 to the negative discrepancies before these values are squared in the calculation of the usual chi-square statistic. If the sample size is large the correction will have little effect on the value of the test statistic.

Appendix A
Statistical Graphics in Medical Investigations

A.1 Introduction

The formal modelling of medical data by any of the techniques described in the ten chapters of this book needs, in practice, to be combined with, or enhanced by, an initial attempt to understand the general characteristics of the data by graphing them in some hopefully useful and informative manner. Graphical displays are also useful when assessing particular aspects of the fit of models. This appendix describes some statistical graphics particularly relevant to medical research.

A.2 Probability plots

Probability plots have been around for a long time, but they remain a useful technique for assessing distributional assumptions, particularly for the residuals from fitting some model or other – several examples have been given in this book. The classic example of such a plot is that for investigating the assumption that a set of data is from a normal distribution; here the ordered sample values, $y_{(1)} \le y_{(2)} \le \ldots \le y_{(n)}$, are plotted against the quantiles of a standard normal distribution, $\Phi^{-1}(p_i)$, where

$$p_i = \frac{i - \frac{1}{2}}{n} \quad \text{and} \quad \Phi(x) = \int_{-\infty}^{x} \frac{1}{\sqrt{2\pi}} e^{-u^2/2} \, du$$

Departures from linearity in the plot indicate that the data do not have a normal distribution.

To illustrate the use of the normal probability plot in particular, and probability plots in general, we shall use the data on survival times of 43 patients suffering from chronic granulocytic leukaemia shown in Table A.1. The normal probability plot of the data shown in Figure A.1 clearly departs from linearity, indicating that the data are not normally distributed. Figure A.2 shows four other probability plots for these data; in Figure A.2(a) an exponential distribution is assessed, and the remaining three plots involve gamma distributions with different shape parameters. The plot for the

Table A.1 Survival times of 43 patients suffering from chronic granulocytic leukaemia, in days from time of diagnosis

7	47	58	74	177	232	273	285	317	429
440	445	455	468	495	497	532	571	579	581
650	702	715	779	881	900	930	968	1077	1109
1314	1334	1367	1534	1712	1784	1877	1886	2045	2056
2260	2429	2509							

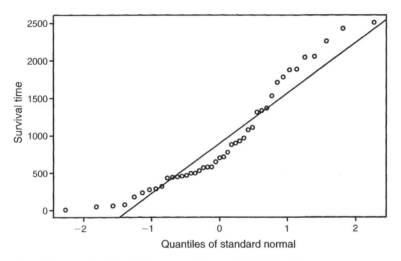

Figure A.1 Normal probability plot for survival times data in Table A.1.

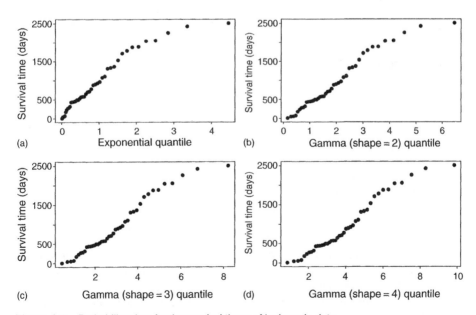

Figure A.2 Probability plots for the survival times of leukaemia data.

exponential distribution looks approximately linear, and this may be a reasonable distribution to assume for the survival times.

When multivariate data are involved, the probability plots described above can be used to examine each variable separately. To use such plots to examine the 'joint' distribution of the variables requires a way of converting the multivariate observation to a single number in some way. For example, in the specific case of assessing a data set for multivariate normality, each q-dimensional observation, x_i, could be transformed into a generalized distance, d_i^2, giving a measure of the separation of the particular observation from the mean vector of the complete sample, $\bar{x}$; d_i^2 is given by

$$d_i^2 = (x_i - \bar{x})' \, S^{-1}(x_i - \bar{x}) \tag{A.1}$$

where S is the sample covariance matrix. If the observations *are* from a multivariate normal distribution, then these distances have approximately a chi-square distribution with q degrees of freedom; plotting the ordered distances against the corresponding quantiles of the appropriate chi-square distribution should lead to a straight line through the origin.

This type of plot can be illustrated on the data in Table A.2, which show the values observed for seven variables during a health survey of paint sprayers in a car assembly plant. The variables are as follows:

HAEMO   – haemoglobin concentration
PCV   – packed cell volume
WBC   – white blood cell count
LYMPHO – lymphocyte count
NEUTRO – neutrophil count
LEAD   – serum lead concentration

The chi-square plot for the data in Table A.2 is shown in Figure A.3. There is a clear departure from linearity caused by six or seven observations being relatively distant from the mean vector of the data. In any analysis of these data it would be wise to identify the relevant observations and decide whether or not they should be excluded.

A.3   Scatterplots and beyond

The simple xy scatterplot has been in use since at least the eighteenth century and has many advantages for an initial exploration of data. Indeed, according to Tufte (1983):

> The relational graphic – in its barest form the scatterplot and its variants – is the greatest of all graphical designs. It links at least two variables encouraging and even imploring the viewer to assess the possible causal relationship between the plotted variables. It confronts causal theories that x causes y with empirical evidence as to the actual relationship between x and y.

To illustrate various aspects of the possible use of scatterplots in medical research, we shall use the data shown in Table A.3, taken with permission from Fisher and van Belle (1993). The data consist of mortality rates due to malignant melanoma of the skin for white males during the period 1950–1969, for each state on the US mainland. Also given are the latitude and longitude of the centre of each state, and a binary variable indicating contiguity to an ocean, where a one indicates contiguity – that is, the state borders one of the oceans. (The population size of each state, also given in Table A.3, will be used later.)

Table A.2   Haematology of paint sprayers

Case	HAEMO	PCV	WBC	LYMPHO	NEUTRO	LEAD
1	13.4	39	4100	14	25	17
2	14.6	46	5000	15	30	20
3	13.5	42	4500	19	21	18
4	15.0	46	4600	23	16	18
5	14.6	44	5100	17	31	19
6	14.0	44	4900	20	24	19
7	16.4	49	4300	21	17	18
8	14.8	44	4400	16	26	29
9	15.2	46	4100	27	13	27
10	15.5	48	8400	34	42	36
11	15.2	48	5600	26	27	22
12	16.9	50	5100	28	17	23
13	14.8	44	4700	24	20	23
14	16.2	45	5600	26	25	19
15	14.7	43	4000	23	13	17
16	14.7	42	3400	9	22	13
17	16.5	45	5400	18	32	17
18	15.4	45	6900	28	36	24
19	15.1	45	4600	17	29	17
20	14.2	46	4200	14	25	28
21	15.9	46	5200	8	34	16
22	16.0	47	4700	25	14	18
23	17.4	50	8600	37	39	17
24	14.3	43	5500	20	31	19
25	14.8	44	4200	15	24	19
26	14.9	43	4300	9	32	17
27	15.5	45	5200	16	30	20
28	14.5	43	3900	18	18	25
29	14.4	45	6000	17	37	23
30	14.6	44	4700	23	21	27
31	15.3	45	7900	43	23	23
32	14.9	45	3400	17	15	24
33	15.8	47	6000	23	32	21
34	14.4	44	7700	31	39	23
35	14.7	46	3700	11	23	23
36	14.8	43	5200	25	19	22
37	15.4	45	6000	30	25	18
38	16.2	50	8100	32	38	18
39	15.0	45	4900	17	26	24
40	15.1	47	6000	22	33	16
41	16.0	46	4600	20	22	22
42	15.3	48	5500	20	23	23
43	14.5	41	6200	20	36	21
44	14.2	41	4900	26	20	20
45	15.0	45	7200	40	25	25
46	14.2	46	5800	22	31	22
47	14.9	45	8400	61	17	17
48	16.2	48	3100	12	15	18
49	14.5	45	4000	20	18	20
50	16.4	49	6900	35	22	24
51	14.7	44	7800	38	34	16

(Continued)

Table A.2   (*Continued*)

Case	HAEMO	PCV	WBC	LYMPHO	NEUTRO	LEAD
52	17.0	52	6300	19	21	16
53	15.4	47	3400	12	19	18
54	13.8	40	4500	19	23	21
55	16.1	47	4600	17	28	20
56	14.6	45	4700	23	22	27
57	15.0	44	5800	14	39	21
58	16.2	47	4100	16	24	18
59	17.0	51	5700	26	29	20
60	14.0	44	4100	16	24	18
61	15.4	46	6200	32	25	16
62	15.6	46	4700	28	16	16
63	15.8	48	4500	24	20	23
64	13.2	38	5300	16	26	20
65	14.9	47	5000	22	25	15
66	14.9	47	3900	15	19	16
67	14.0	45	5200	23	25	17
68	16.1	47	4300	19	22	22
69	14.7	46	6800	35	25	18
70	17.0	51	6300	42	19	15
71	17.0	51	6300	42	19	15
72	15.2	45	4600	21	22	18
73	15.2	43	5600	25	28	17
74	13.8	41	6300	25	27	15
75	14.8	43	6400	36	24	18
76	16.1	47	5200	18	28	25
77	15.0	43	6300	22	34	17
78	16.2	46	6000	25	25	24
79	14.8	44	3900	9	25	14
80	17.2	44	4100	12	27	18
81	17.2	48	5000	25	19	25
82	14.6	43	5500	22	31	19
83	14.4	44	4300	20	20	15
84	15.4	48	5700	29	26	24
85	16.0	52	4100	21	15	22
86	15.0	45	5000	27	18	20
87	14.8	44	5700	29	23	23
88	15.4	43	3300	10	20	15
89	16.0	47	6100	32	23	26
90	14.8	43	5100	18	31	19
91	13.8	41	8100	52	24	17
92	14.7	43	5200	24	24	17
93	14.6	44	9899	69	28	18
94	13.6	42	6100	24	30	15
95	14.5	44	4800	14	29	15
96	14.3	39	5000	25	20	19
97	15.3	45	4000	19	19	16
98	16.4	49	6000	34	22	17
99	14.8	44	4500	22	18	25
100	16.6	48	4700	17	27	20
101	16.0	49	7000	36	28	18
102	15.5	46	6600	30	33	13
103	14.3	46	5700	26	20	21

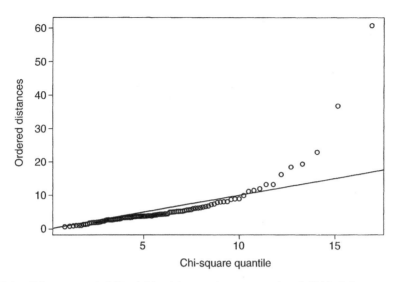

Figure A.3 Chi-square probability plot for data on paint sprayers given in Table A.2.

The two simple scatterplots in Figure A.4 show annual mortality plotted against latitude and longitude. Figure A.4(a) shows a very clear decline in mortality with increasing latitude, as would be expected. On the other hand, Figure A.4(b) demonstrates that there is essentially no relationship between longitude and mortality. The two scatterplots can be enhanced by adding both linear and locally weighted regression fits to highlight the trend (or lack of it) in both plots – see Figure A.5.

It is also useful to enhance the basic scatterplots with labels identifying ocean and non-ocean states; these are given in Figure A.6. Figure A.6(a) clearly demonstrates the higher mortality rates associated with ocean states, for the same latitude; it also suggests that the decline in mortality with latitude is approximately the same for both ocean and non-ocean states.

Although the scatterplot is a primary data-analytic tool for assessing the relationship between a pair of continuous variables, it is often difficult to judge whether or not the variables are independent – a random scatter of points is hard for the human eye to judge. Consequently it is often helpful to augment the scatterplot with an auxiliary display in which independence is itself manifested in a characteristic manner. The *chi-plot* suggested by Fisher and Switzer (1985, 2001) is designed to address the problem. A chi-plot is a scatterplot of the pairs (λ_i, χ_i),

$$|\lambda_i| < 4 \left\{ \frac{1}{n-1} - \frac{1}{2} \right\}^2$$

where

$$\chi_i = \frac{H_i - F_i G_i}{\left\{ F_i (1 - F_i) G_i (1 - G_i) \right\}^{1/2}} \tag{A.2}$$

Table A.3 Mortality rates due to malignant melanoma in the USA

State	Mortality	Latitude	Longitude	Population size (millions)	Ocean state (1 = yes, 0 = no)
Alabama	219	33.0	87.0	3.46	1
Arizona	160	34.5	112.0	1.61	0
Arkansas	170	35.0	92.5	1.96	0
California	182	37.5	119.5	18.60	1
Colorado	149	39.0	105.5	1.97	0
Connecticut	159	41.8	72.8	2.83	1
Delaware	200	39.0	75.5	0.50	1
Florida	197	28.0	82.0	5.80	1
Georgia	214	33.0	83.5	4.36	1
Idaho	116	44.5	114.0	0.69	0
Illinois	124	40.0	89.5	10.64	0
Indiana	128	40.2	86.2	4.88	0
Iowa	128	42.2	93.8	2.76	0
Kansas	166	38.5	98.5	2.23	0
Kentucky	147	37.8	85.0	3.18	0
Louisiana	190	31.2	91.8	3.53	1
Maine	117	45.2	69.0	0.99	1
Maryland	162	39.0	765.0	3.52	1
Massachusetts	143	42.2	71.8	5.35	1
Michigan	117	43.5	84.5	8.22	0
Minnesota	116	46.0	94.5	3.55	0
Mississippi	207	32.8	90.0	2.32	1
Missouri	131	38.5	92.0	4.50	0
Montana	109	47.0	110.5	0.71	0
Nebraska	122	41.5	99.5	1.48	0
Nevada	191	39.0	117.0	0.44	0
New Hampshire	129	43.8	71.5	0.67	1
New Jersey	159	40.2	74.5	6.77	1
New Mexico	141	35.0	106.0	1.03	0
New York	152	43.0	75.5	18.07	1
North Carolina	199	35.5	79.5	4.91	1
North Dakota	115	47.5	100.5	0.65	0
Ohio	131	40.2	82.8	10.24	0
Oklahoma	182	35.5	97.2	2.48	0
Oregon	136	44.0	120.5	1.90	1
Pennsylvania	132	40.8	77.8	11.52	0
Rhode Island	137	41.8	71.5	0.92	1
South Carolina	178	33.8	81.0	2.54	1
South Dakota	86	44.8	100.0	0.70	0
Tennessee	186	36.0	86.2	3.84	0
Texas	229	31.5	98.0	10.55	1
Utah	142	39.5	111.5	0.99	0
Vermont	153	44.0	72.5	0.40	1
Virginia	166	37.5	78.5	4.46	1
Washington	117	47.5	121.0	2.99	1
West Virginia	136	38.8	80.8	1.81	0
Wisconsin	110	44.5	90.2	4.14	0
Wyoming	134	43.0	107.5	0.34	0

Source: Taken with permission of the publishers, Wiley, from Fisher and van Belle (1993).

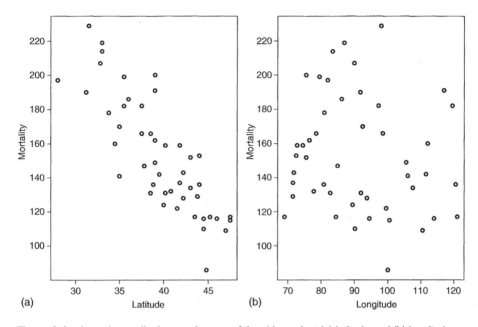

Figure A.4   Annual mortality from melanoma of the skin against (a) latitude and (b) longitude.

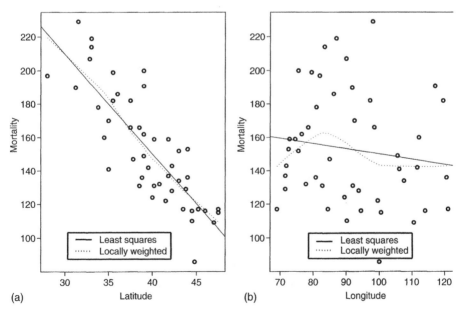

Figure A.5   Scatterplot of (a) latitude and (b) longitude against mortality from melanoma of the skin, enhanced with least-squares and locally weighted regression fits.

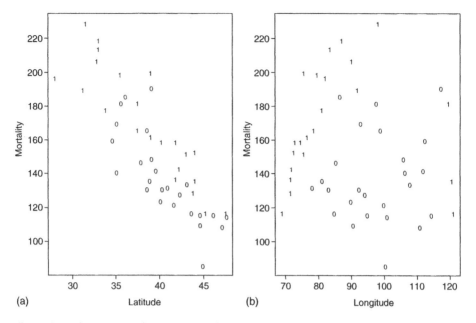

Figure A.6   Scatterplot of (a) latitude and (b) longitude against mortality from melanoma of the skin, enhanced with labels for ocean (1) and non-ocean states (0).

$$\lambda_i = 4S_i \max\left\{\left(F_i - \frac{1}{2}\right)^2, \left(G_i - \frac{1}{2}\right)^2\right\} \tag{A.3}$$

and

$$H_i = \frac{1}{n-1}\sum_{j\neq i} I(x_j \leq x_i, y_j \leq y_i) \tag{A.4}$$

$$F_i = \frac{1}{n-1}\sum_{j\neq i} I(x_j \leq x_i) \tag{A.5}$$

$$G_i = \frac{1}{n-1}\sum_{j\neq i} I(y_j \leq y_i) \tag{A.6}$$

$$S_i = \text{sign}\left\{\left(F_i - \frac{1}{2}\right)\left(G_i - \frac{1}{2}\right)\right\} \tag{A.7}$$

where sign(x) is $+1$ if x is positive, 0 if x is zero and -1 if x is negative; $I(A)$ is the indicator function for the event A, that is, if A is true then $I(A) = 1$, if A is not true then $I(A) = 0$.

To illustrate the chi-plot we shall apply it to the mortality data in Table A.3. Figure A.7 shows mortality plotted against latitude and the corresponding chi-plot, and Figure A.8 shows the corresponding pair of diagrams for longitude and mortality. The lack of relationship between mortality and longitude is strikingly clear from the chi-plot in Figure A.8.

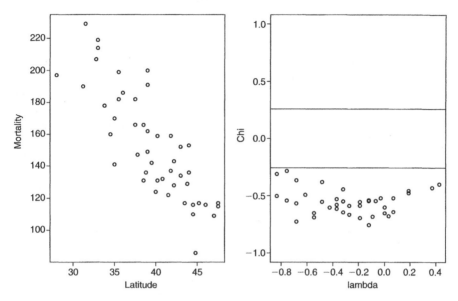

Figure A.7   Scatterplot and chi-plot of mortality and latitude.

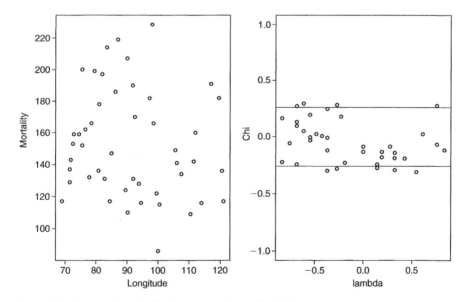

Figure A.8   Scatterplot and chi-plot of mortality and longitude.

A further helpful addition to the scatterplot is the two-dimensional analogue of the boxplot for univariate data, known as the *bivariate boxplot* (Goldberg and Iglewicz, 1992); this may be useful in indicating the distributional properties of the data and in identifying possible outliers. The bivariate boxplot is based on calculating 'robust' measures of location, scale and correlation; it consists essentially of a pair of concentric ellipses, of which one (the 'hinge') includes 50% of the data and the other (the 'fence') delineates potential troublesome outliers. In addition, resistant regression lines of both y on x and x on y are shown, with their intersection showing the bivariate location estimator. The acute angle between the regression lines will be small for a large absolute value of correlations and large for a small one. Details of the construction of a bivariate boxplot are as follows:

- To draw the elliptical fence and hinge, location (T_x^*, T_y^*), scale (S_x^*, S_y^*) and correlation (R^*) estimators are needed and, in addition, a constant D that regulates the distance of the fence from the hinge. In general $D = 7$ is recommended since this corresponds to an approximate 99% confidence bound on a single observation.
- In general, robust estimators of location, scale and correlation are recommended since they are better at handling data with outliers or with density or shape differing moderately from the elliptical bivariate normal. Goldberg and Iglewicz (1992) discuss a number of possibilities.
- To draw the bivariate boxplot, first calculate the median E_m and the maximum $E_{\max}$ of the standardized errors, E_i, which are essentially the generalized distances of each point from the centre (T_x^*, T_y^*). Specifically, the E_i are defined by

$$E_i = \sqrt{\frac{X_{si}^2 + Y_{si}^2 - 2R^* X_{si} Y_{si}}{1 - R^{*2}}}$$

where $X_{si} = (X_i - T_x^*)/S_x^*$ is the standardized X_i value and Y_{si} is similarly defined.

- Then

$$E_m = \text{median}\{E_i : i = 1, 2, ..., n\}$$

and

$$E_{\max} = \max\{E_i : E_i^2 < DE_m^2\}$$

- To draw the hinge, let

$$R_1 = E_m \sqrt{\frac{1 + R^*}{2}}, \qquad R_2 = E_m \sqrt{\frac{1 - R^*}{2}}$$

- For $\theta = 0$ to 360 in steps of 2, 3, 4 or 5 degrees, let

$$\Theta_1 = R_1 \cos\theta,$$
$$\Theta_2 = R_2 \sin\theta,$$
$$X = T_x^* + (\Theta_1 + \Theta_2)S_x^*,$$
$$Y = T_y^* + (\Theta_1 - \Theta_2)S_y^*$$

- Finally, plot X, Y.

To illustrate the use of a bivariate boxplot we shall use the mortality and latitude variables in Table A.3, after the addition of a new observation with latitude 30 and mortality 250. A scatterplot of the amended data is shown in Figure A.9. It is difficult to identify any possible outliers in this plot. In Figure A.10 the scatterplot is enhanced by the bivariate boxplot of the two variables; the new observation is now indicated as a likely outlier.

The basic scatterplot can only accommodate two variables, but other variable values can be displayed on the plot in a variety of ways. The simplest is perhaps by what is known as the *bubbleplot*; here two variables are used to form the scatterplot, and the

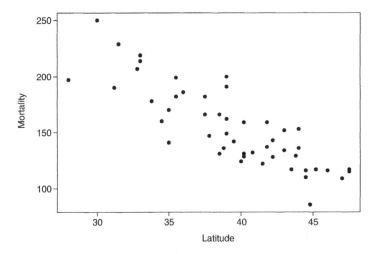

Figure A.9   Scatterplot of mortality and latitude with one added observation.

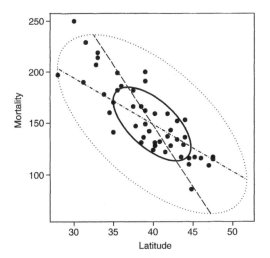

Figure A.10   Scatterplot enhanced with bivariate boxplot for new mortality and latitude data.

values of a third variable are represented by circles with radii proportional to those values, centred on the appropriate point in the scatterplot. A bubbleplot of latitude, longitude and mortality is shown in Figure A.11.

Other possibilities for representing three-dimensional data are illustrated in Figures A.12 and A.13; in Figure A.14 a 'smooth' surface has been fitted to the mortality rates to highlight how they change with changes in latitude and longitude.

An important parameter of a scatterplot that can greatly influence our ability to recognize patterns is the *aspect ratio*, the physical length of the vertical axis divided by that of the horizontal axis. Most computer packages produce plots with an aspect ratio near 1, but this is not always the best value. To illustrate how changing this characteristic of a scatterplot can help understand what the data are trying to tell us, we shall use the example given by Cook and Weisberg (1994) involving monthly US births per thousand population for the years 1940–1948. The data are given in Table A.4, and a scatterplot of the birth rates against month with an aspect ratio of 1 is shown in

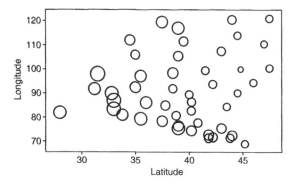

Figure A.11   Bubbleplot of mortality against latitude and longitude.

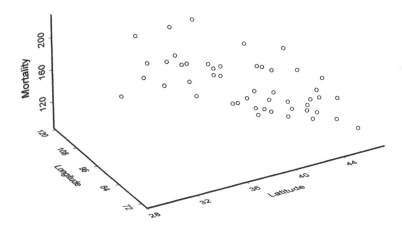

Figure A.12   Three-dimensional scatterplot of mortality from melanoma of the skin against latitude and longitude.

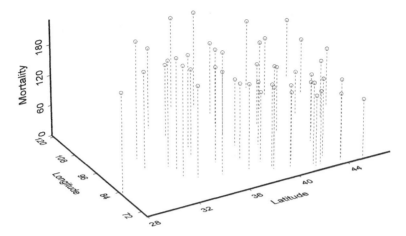

Figure A.13 Three-dimensional scatterplot with drop lines for mortality from melanoma of the skin against latitude and longitude.

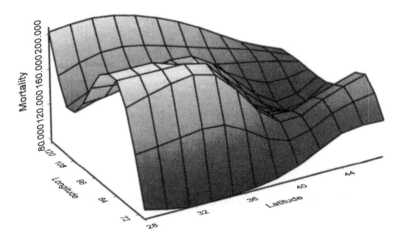

Figure A.14 Three-dimensional scatterplot with fitted surface for mortality from melanoma of the skin against latitude and longitude.

Figure A.15. The plot shows that the US birth rate was increasing between 1940 and 1943, decreasing between 1943 and 1946, rapidly increasing during 1946, and then decreasing again during 1947–1978. As Cook and Weisberg comment:

> These trends seem to deliver an interesting history lesson since the US involvement in World War II started in 1942 and troops began returning home during the first part of 1945, about nine months before the rapid increase in the birth rate.

Now let us see what happens when the data are replotted with an aspect ratio of 0.3; the result appears in Figure A.16. The new plot displays many peaks and troughs and suggests perhaps some minor within-year trends in addition to the global trends apparent

Table A.4 US monthly birth rates between 1940 and 1943 (read along rows for temporal sequence)

1890	1957	1925	1885	1896	1934	2036	2069	2060
1922	1854	1852	1952	2011	2015	1971	1883	2070
2221	2173	2105	1962	1951	1975	2092	2148	2114
2013	1986	2088	2218	2312	2462	2455	2357	2309
2398	2400	2331	2222	2156	2256	2352	2371	2356
2211	2108	2069	2123	2147	2050	1977	1993	2134
2275	2262	2194	2109	2114	2086	2089	2097	2036
1957	1953	2039	2116	2134	2142	2023	1972	1942
1931	1980	1977	1972	2017	2161	2468	2691	2890
2913	2940	2870	2911	2832	2774	2568	2574	2641
2691	2698	2701	2596	2503	2424			

Source: Cook and Weisberg (1994).

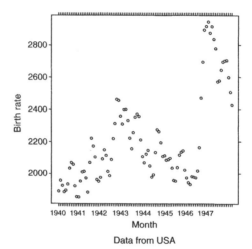

Figure A.15 US birth rate against year plotted with aspect ratio 1.0.

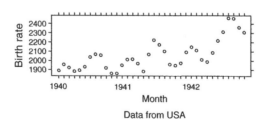

Figure A.16 US birth rate against year plotted with aspect ratio 0.3.

in Figure A.15. A clearer picture is obtained by plotting only a part of the data, as is done in Figure A.17 for the years 1940–1943. Now a within-year cycle is clearly apparent, with the lowest within-year birth rate at the beginning of the summer and the highest occurring in the autumn.

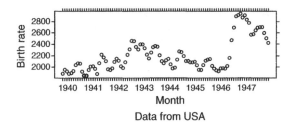

Figure A.17   US birth rate against year (1940–1947) with aspect ratio 0.3.

Examination of scatterplots often centres on assessing density patterns such as clusters, gaps or outliers. But humans are not particularly good at visualizing point density, and some type of density estimate added to the scatterplot is often helpful. Density estimation is described in Silverman (1986), but no details are given here; instead we shall just give an example using the data on birth and death rates for 69 countries shown in Table A.5. A scatterplot of the data, enhanced by a contour plot of the estimated bivariate density, is shown in Figure A.18. The plot gives some evidence of two modes in the data corresponding largely to countries in the West and in the Third World.

A.4   Scatterplot matrices

A scatterplot matrix is defined as a square, symmetric grid of bivariate scatterplots; it acts as a convenient way of arranging all the pairwise scatterplots in a set of multivariate data with, say, q variables. The grid has q rows and q columns, each one corresponding to a different variable. Each of the grid's cells shows a scatterplot of two variables. Variable j is plotted against variable i in the ijth cell and the same variables appear in cell ji with the x and y axes of the scatterplots interchanged. The reason for including both the upper and lower triangles of the grid, despite the apparent redundancy, is that it enables a row and column to be visually scanned to see one variable against all others, with the scales for the one variable lined up along the horizontal or the vertical.

The use of a scatterplot matrix can be illustrated on the data shown in Table A.6, giving the nutrients in 3 ounces of various foodstuffs. The basic scatterplot matrix of the data is shown in Figure A.19. The relationships between several pairs of the nutrients appear complex and are certainly not linear. In addition, there appear to be a number of outliers in some of the scatterplots. Identifying which of the foodstuffs correspond to these outliers can be made by plotting the codes for each of them – see Figure A.20. Clams, both raw and canned, are now seen to be the most obvious outliers – both are extremely high in iron. The possible nonlinearity of the relationship between some pairs of nutrients can be highlighted, by including both a linear fit and a locally weighted fit on each panel of the scatterplot matrix – see Figure A.21. On some panels, for example energy and protein, the linear and locally weighted fits differ considerably. On others, for example fat and energy, they are almost identical.

Table A.5   Birth and death rates for 69 countries

Country	Birth	Death	Country	Birth	Death
alg	36.4	14.6	con	37.3	8.0
egy	42.1	15.3	gha	55.8	25.6
ict	56.1	33.1	mag	41.8	15.8
mor	46.1	18.7	tun	41.7	10.1
cam	41.4	19.7	cey	35.8	8.5
chi	34.0	11.0	tai	36.3	6.1
hkg	32.1	5.5	ind	20.9	8.8
ids	27.7	10.2	irq	20.5	3.9
isr	25.0	6.2	jap	17.3	7.0
jor	46.3	6.4	kor	14.8	5.7
mal	33.5	6.4	mog	39.2	11.2
phl	28.4	7.1	syr	26.2	4.3
tha	34.8	7.9	vit	23.4	5.1
can	24.8	7.8	cra	49.9	8.5
dmr	33.0	8.4	gut	47.7	17.3
hon	46.6	9.7	mex	45.1	10.5
nic	42.9	7.1	pan	10.1	8.0
usa	21.7	9.6	arg	21.8	8.1
bol	17.4	5.8	bra	45.0	13.5
chl	33.6	11.8	clo	44.0	11.7
ecu	44.2	13.5	per	27.7	8.2
urg	22.5	7.8	ven	42.8	6.7
aus	18.8	12.8	bel	17.1	12.7
brt	18.2	12.2	bul	16.4	8.2
cze	16.9	9.5	dem	17.6	19.8
fin	18.1	9.2	fra	18.2	11.7
gmy	18.0	12.5	gre	17.4	7.8
hun	13.1	9.9	irl	22.3	11.9
ity	19.0	10.2	net	20.9	8.0
now	17.5	10.0	pol	19.0	7.5
pog	23.5	10.8	rom	15.7	8.3
spa	21.5	9.1	swe	14.8	10.1
swz	18.9	9.6	rus	21.2	7.2
yug	21.4	8.9	ast	21.6	8.7
nzl	25.5	8.8			

A.5   Coplots and trellis graphics

The conditioning plot or coplot is a potentially powerful visualization tool for studying how, say, a response variable depends on two or more explanatory variables. In essence, such plots display the bivariate relationship between two variables while holding constant (or 'conditioning upon') the values of one or more other variables. As an example, Figure A.22 shows a coplot of mortality versus latitude conditioned on population size. In this diagram, the panel at the top of the figure is known as the *given* panel; the panels below are *dependence* panels. Each rectangle in the given panel specifies a range of values of population size. On a corresponding dependence panel, mortality is plotted against latitude for those states whose population sizes lie in the particular interval. To match population size intervals to dependence panels, the latter are examined in order from left to right in the bottom row and then again from left to right in subsequent rows. The association between higher values of mortality

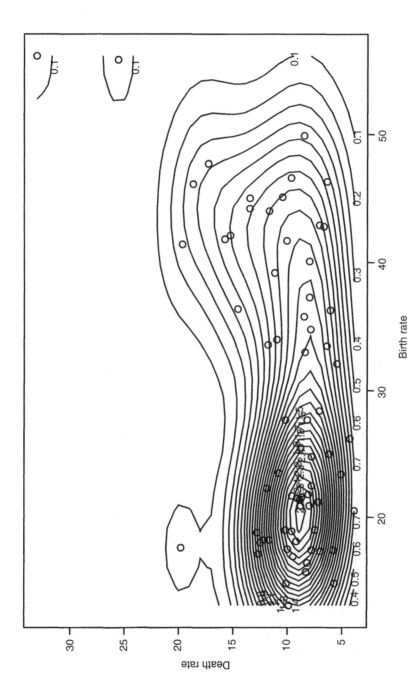

Figure A.18 Contour plot of estimated bivariate density for birth/death rate data.

Table A.6   Nutrients in food data

	Energy (kcal)	Protein (g)	Fat (g)	Calcium (mg)	Iron (mg)
BB Beef, braised	340	20	28	9	2.6
HR Hamburger	245	21	17	9	2.7
BR Beef roast	420	15	39	7	2.0
BS Beef, steak	375	19	32	9	2.5
BC Beef, canned	180	22	10	17	3.7
CB Chicken, broiled	115	20	3	8	1.4
CC Chicken, canned	170	25	7	12	1.5
BH Beef, heart	160	26	5	14	5.9
LL Lamb leg, roast	265	20	20	9	2.6
LS Lamb shoulder, roast	300	18	25	9	2.3
HS Smoked ham	340	20	28	9	2.5
PR Pork roast	340	19	29	9	2.5
PS Pork simmered	355	19	30	9	2.4
BT Beef tongue	205	18	14	7	2.5
VC Veal cutlet	185	23	9	9	2.7
FB Bluefish, baked	135	22	4	25	0.6
AR Clams, raw	70	11	1	82	6.0
AC Clams, canned	45	7	1	74	5.4
TC Crabmeat, canned	90	14	2	38	0.8
HF Haddock, fried	135	16	5	15	0.5
MB Mackerel, broiled	200	19	13	5	1.0
MC Mackerel, canned	155	16	9	157	1.8
PF Perch, fried	195	16	11	14	1.3
SC Salmon, canned	120	17	5	159	0.7
DC Sardines, canned	180	22	9	367	2.5
UC Tuna, canned	170	25	7	7	1.2
RC Shrimp, canned	110	23	1	98	2.6

and lower values of latitude (and vice versa), is seen to hold for all levels of population size.

Conditional graphical displays are simple examples of a more general scheme known as *trellis graphics* (Becker and Cleveland, 1994). This is an approach to examining high-dimensional structure in data by means of one-, two- and three-dimensional graphs. The problem addressed is how observations of one or more variables depend on the observations of the other variables. The essential feature of this approach is the multiple conditioning that allows some type of plot to be displayed for different values of a given variable (or variables). The aim is to help in understanding both the structure of the data and how well proposed models describe the structure. An excellent recent example of the application of trellis graphics is given in Verbyla *et al.* (1999). To illustrate the possibilities we shall return to the mortality from skin melanoma data; Figures A.23–A.25 show three trellis displays. Figure A.23 gives a scatterplot matrix of the three variables mortality, latitude and longitude, conditional on population size. Figure A.24 shows a bubble plot of mortality, latitude and longitude, conditioned on both population size and ocean contiguity. For states with low population size, latitude and mortality do not have the clear relationship found overall. Figure A.25 shows fitted bivariate surfaces of mortality, latitude and longitude, conditioned on population size.

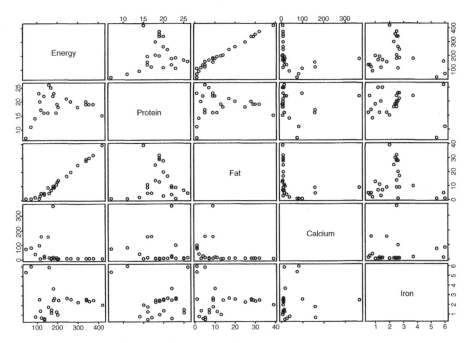

Figure A.19 Scatterplot matrix of nutrients in food.

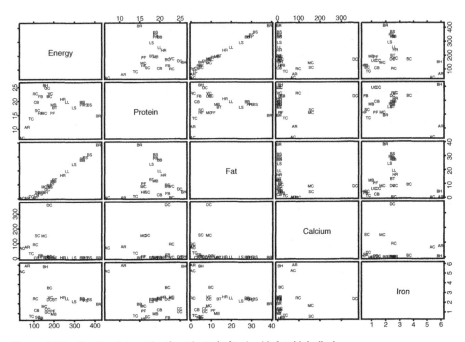

Figure A.20 Scatterplot matrix of nutrients in food, with food labelled.

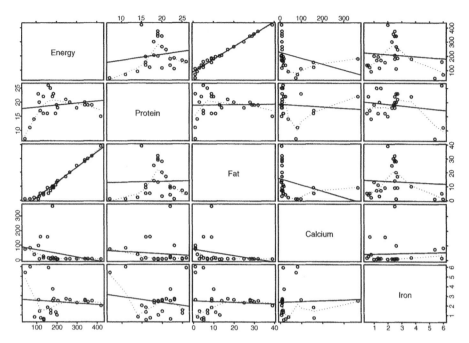

Figure A.21   Scatterplot matrix of nutrients in food, showing least-squares and locally weighted regression fits.

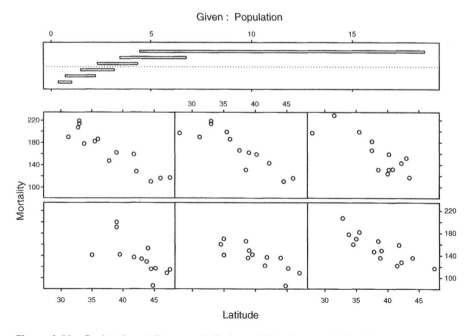

Figure A.22   Coplot of mortality versus latitude conditioned on population size.

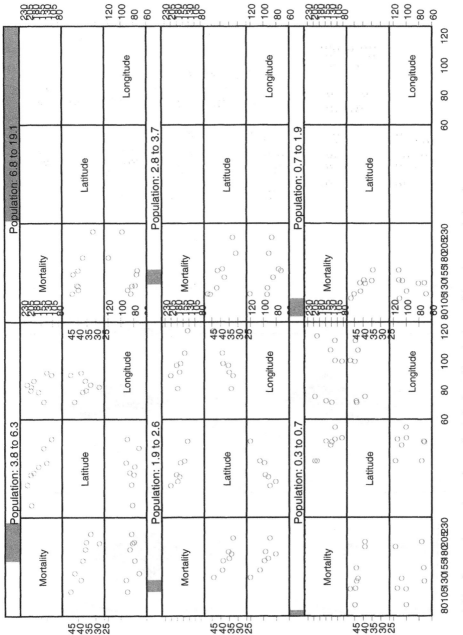

Figure A.23 Scatterplot matrices of mortality, latitude and longitude conditioned on population size.

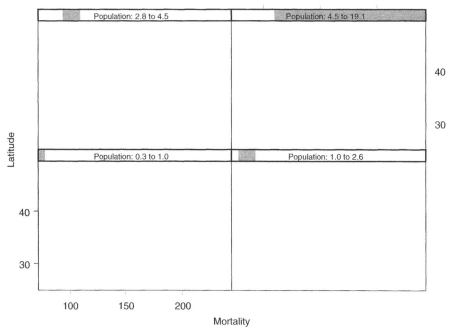

Figure A.24 Bubbleplots of mortality, latitude and longitude, conditioned on population size and ocean state.

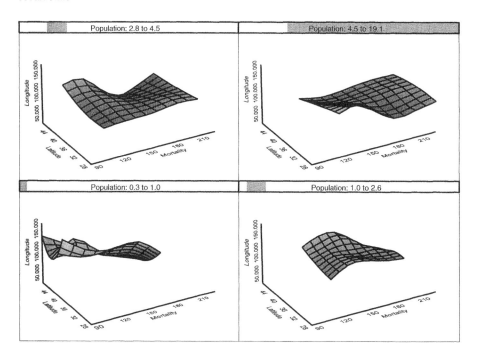

Figure A.25 Bivariate surfaces for mortality latitude and longitude conditioned on population size.

Trellis graphics are a potentially very exciting and powerful tool for the exploration of data from medical studies. But a word of caution is perhaps in order. With data sets of small or moderate size, the number of observations in each panel may be too few to make the panel graphic helpful.

Software

All the graphs given in this appendix were constructed using S-PLUS, but many could no doubt have been derived from other packages. The graphics facilities of S-PLUS are, however, extremely powerful and flexible. More examples of using S-PLUS to construct graphical displays are given in Everitt and Rabe-Hesketh (2001) and Everitt (2001).

Appendix B
Answers to Selected Exercises

Chapter 1

1.1 The following analysis of deviance tables suggest that a model including only *weight* and *age* is necessary.

Model	df	Resid. dev.	Test	df	Deviance
1. weight	18	54.53			
2. weight + age	17	4.82	age	1	49.70

Model	df	Resid. dev.	Test	df	Deviance
1. weight + age	17	4.82			
2. weight + age + ba	16	3.06	ba	1	1.77

Model	df	Resid. dev.	Test	df	Deviance
1. weight + age + ba	16	3.06			
2. weight + age + ba + stress	15	2.84	stress	1	0.22

Model	df	Resid. dev.	Test	df	Deviance
1. weight + age + ba + stress	15	2.84			
2. weight + age + ba + stress + time + pulse	13	2.16	time + pulse	2	0.68

1.3 The results from fitting a model including log(acid) and all other explanatory variables are as follows:

Covariates	Estimated regression coefficient	Standard error	Coeff./SE
Age	−0.09	0.06	−1.52
Log(acid)	2.65	1.20	2.20
X-ray	1.65	0.81	2.04
Size	2.01	0.82	2.45
Grade	0.40	0.81	0.49

The conclusions are largely the same as from the results given in Table 1.4.
   Including interactions in the model gives the following results:

Covariates	Estimated regression coefficient	Standard error	Coeff./SE
Age	−0.12	0.07	−1.61
Grade	4.75	2.33	2.04
Log(acid)	1.93	1.50	1.29
X-ray	1.72	0.92	1.86
Size	3.24	1.18	2.74
Grade × log(acid)	5.14	4.06	1.26
Size × grade	−3.32	1.92	1.74

Neither interaction appears of great importance.

Chapter 2

2.1 Allowing a time × dose interaction in the random intercept and slope model for the data gives the following results:

Covariates	Estimated regression coefficient	Standard error	Coeff./SE
Time	0.08	0.032	2.71
Dose	−0.05	0.043	−1.26
Age	−0.02	0.012	−1.38
Duration	−0.01	0.006	−1.58
Time × dose	0.001	0.001	0.39

There is no evidence of a time × dose interaction.
   Now allowing a quadratic effect of time into the original random intercept and slope model leads to the following:

Covariates	Estimated regression coefficient	Standard error	Coeff./SE
Time	0.064	0.020	3.20
Time^2	0.001	0.001	1.98
Dose	−0.045	0.036	−1.24
Age	−0.017	0.012	−1.38
Duration	−0.009	0.006	−1.58

There is perhaps some evidence of the need for a quadratic effect of time.

2.4 The consequences of this model for the variance–covariance structure of the repeated measures are:

$$\text{Var}(y_{ij}) = \sigma_{u_1}^2 + 2t_j\,\sigma_{u_1 u_2} + t_j^2\,\sigma_{u_2}^2 + \sigma^2$$

$$\text{Cov}(y_{ij}, y_{ij'}) = \sigma_{u_1}^2 + (t_j + t_{j'})\,\sigma_{u_1 u_2} + t_j t_{j'}\sigma_{u_2}^2, \quad t \neq t'$$

2.6 The results equivalent to those given in Table 2.15 assuming an identity link function and Gaussian errors are as follows:

Covariates	Estimated regression coefficient	Standard error	Coeff./SE
Time	−0.24	0.23	−1.05
Age	0.19	0.08	2.20
Treat	−0.70	1.04	−0.67
BL	0.36	0.02	18.24

The conclusions would be quite different.

Chapter 3

3.1 Adding treatment group to the model gives the following results:

Covariates	Estimated regression coefficient	Standard error	Coeff./SE
Previous value	0.010	0.005	2.12
Treatment group	−0.164	0.355	−0.46

3.2 The results are as follows:

Covariates	Estimated regression coefficient	Standard error	Coeff./SE
(a) Unconditional means			
Group	35.35	4.14	8.53
Time	0.21	0.02	12.76
(b) LOCF			
Group	28.53	6.10	4.68
Time	0.16	0.01	10.39

Chapter 4

4.4 Results of fitting a logistic additive model to the ESR data and comparison with a linear logistic model:

Term	df	df. npar.	Chi-square	p-value
s(Fibrinogen)	1	2.9	4.31	0.214
s(Gamma)	1	2.9	2.61	0.429

Model	Terms	df	Resid. Dev.
logistic regression	Fibrinogen + Gamma	29	22.97
GAM	s(Fibrinogen) + s(Gamma)	23.27	11.09

Chapter 5

5.2 The resulting tree is as follows:

```
node), split, n, deviance, yval, (yprob)
      * denotes terminal node

 1) root 189 235.0 ge2.5 ( 0.688 0.3120 )
    2) smoke:ns 115 130.0 ge2.5 ( 0.748 0.2520 )
       4) race:white 44  26.8 ge2.5 ( 0.909 0.0909 ) *
       5) race:black,other 71  92.1 ge2.5 ( 0.648 0.3520 )
         10) race:black 16  19.9 ge2.5 ( 0.688 0.3120 ) *
         11) race:other 55  72.1 ge2.5 ( 0.636 0.3640 ) *
    3) smoke:s 74  99.9 ge2.5 ( 0.595 0.4050 )
       6) race:black 10  13.5 le2.5 ( 0.400 0.6000 ) *
       7) race:white,other 64  84.7 ge2.5 ( 0.625 0.3750 )
         14) race:white 52  68.3 ge2.5 ( 0.635 0.3650 ) *
         15) race:other 12  16.3 ge2.5 ( 0.583 0.4170 ) *
```

5.3 The results for all explanatory variables are as follows:

```
node), split, n, deviance, yval, (yprob)
      * denotes terminal node

 1) root 53 69.20 Absence ( 0.642 0.3580 )
    2) ACID<0.665 28 23.00 Absence ( 0.857 0.1430 )
       4) AGE<58.5 11 12.90 Absence ( 0.727 0.2730 )
          8) AGE<54.5 6  5.41 Absence ( 0.833 0:1670 ) *
          9) AGE>54.5 5  6.73 Absence ( 0.600 0.4000 ) *
       5) AGE>58.5 17  7.61 Absence ( 0.941 0.0588 )
         10) ACID<0.495 8  6.03 Absence ( 0.875 0.1250 ) *
         11) ACID>0.495 9  0.00 Absence ( 1.000 0.0000 ) *
    3) ACID>0.665 25 33.70 Presence ( 0.400 0.6000 )
       6) SIZE:Small 10 12.20 Absence ( 0.700 0.3000 )
         12) ACID<0.825 5  5.00 Absence ( 0.800 0.2000 ) *
         13) ACID>0.825 5  6.73 Absence ( 0.600 0.4000 ) *
       7) SIZE:Large 15 15.00 Presence ( 0.200 0.8000 )
         14) XRAY:Negative 8 10.60 Presence ( 0.375 0.6250 ) *
         15) XRAY:Positive 7  0.00 Presence ( 0.000 1.0000 ) *
```

The plotted tree is shown in Figure B.1, and the plot of deviance against size is shown in Figure B.2. The tree of size 2 is simply:

$$\text{ACID} > 0.665 \quad \text{Presence of nodal involvement}$$
$$\text{ACID} < 0.665 \quad \text{Absence of nodal involvement}$$

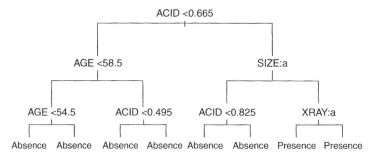

Figure B.1   Classification tree for prostate cancer data.

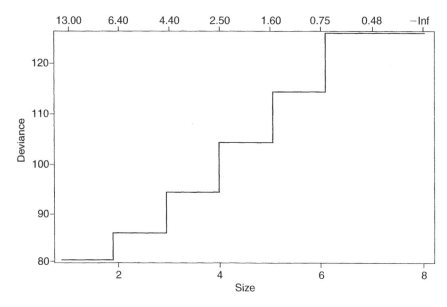

Figure B.2   Plot of deviance against size for prostate cancer trees.

Chapter 6

6.1 Fitting a model including only the two explanatory variables *Size* and *Gleason* gives a log-likelihood value of -11.77; adding the variables *Treatment, Age* and *Haem* increases the log-likelihood to -11.09. This suggests that only *Size* and *Gleason* are needed, although further investigation is necessary to see if both are required.

Chapter 7

7.2 Compare the log-likelihoods of competing models; for example, for the frailty model described in the text including all explanatory variables, the associated log-likelihood is -157.29. Allowing, say, a sex $\times$ *gn* interaction in the model increases the log-likelihood to -155.69. There is no strong evidence that such an interaction is necessary.

Chapter 8

8.2 The calculation of log(relative risk) for each study and its standard error is as follows:

Study	Aspirin		Placebo		Relative risk (rr)[†]	Log of rr(L(rr))[‡]	Standard error of L(rr)[‡]	W = 1/SE² (L(rr))
	n_1	Death rate (p_1)	n_2	Death rate (p_2)				
1	615	0.0797	624	0.1074	1.3476	0.2983	0.1791	31.18
2	759	0.0580	771	0.0830	1.4310	0.3584	0.1891	27.97
3	832	0.1226	850	0.1482	1.2088	0.1896	0.1240	65.04
4	317	0.1009	309	0.1230	1.2190	0.1980	0.2262	19.54
5	810	0.1049	406	0.1281	1.2212	0.1998	0.1652	36.64
6	2267	0.1085	2257	0.0970	0.8940	−0.1120	0.0880	129.13
7	8587	0.1828	8600	0.2000	1.0941	0.0899	0.0314	1014.24

[†]$rr5\ p_2/p_1$.

[‡]$SE_{(L(rr))} = \left(\dfrac{1 - p_1}{n_1 p_1} + \dfrac{1 - p_2}{n_2 p_2} \right)^{1/2}$.

The fixed effects model gives an estimate of 0.0903 with standard error of 0.0275. The random effects model gives an estimate of 0.1135 with standard error of 0.0557. The results of the sensitivity analysis are as follows:

Effect estimate	p-value	95% CI	Pr(Select/V_{min})	Pr(Select/V_{max})	Estimated no. of studies
0.1064	0.047	0.095, 0.2113	1.00	1.00	7
0.843	0.114	−0.0203, 0.1889	0.99	0.80	8
0.0722	0.805	−0.5012, 0.6457	0.80	0.50	12
0.01770	0.860	−0.1796, 0.2150	0.50	0.30	20
0.01733	0.852	−0.1644, 0.1990	0.40	0.10	54
0.01801	0.844	−0.1615, 0.1976	0.20	0.01	456

Chapter 10

10.1 The first two equations in (10.3) remain the same but the third becomes

$$\hat{\Sigma}_c = \frac{1}{n} \sum_{i=1}^{n} \mathbf{x}_i \mathbf{x}_i' - \sum \hat{p}_k \hat{\mu}_k \hat{\mu}_k'$$

where Σ_c is the assumed common variance–covariance matrix.

References

Altman, D.G. (1991). *Practical Statistics for Medical Research*. Chapman & Hall, London.

Altman, D.G. and De Stavola, B.L. (1994). Practical problems in fitting a proportional hazards model to data with updated measurements of the covariates. *Statistics in Medicine* **13**, 301–341.

Andrews, D. and Herzberg, A. (1985). *Data*. Academic Press, New York.

Antman, E.M., Lau, J., Kupelnick, B., Mosteller, F. and Chalmers, T.C. (1992). A comparison of results of meta-analysis of randomized controlled trials and recommendations of clinical experts: treatments for myocardial infarction. *Journal of the American Medical Association* **268**, 240–248.

Aspirin Myocardial Infarction Study Research Group (1980). Aspirin Myocardial Infarction Study Research Group. A randomized controlled trial of aspirin in persons recovered from myocardial infarction. *Journal of the American Medical Association* **243**, 661–669.

Bailey, K.R. (1987). Inter-study differences: how should they influence the interpretation and analysis of results? *Statistics in Medicine* **6**, 351–358.

Becker, R.A. and Cleveland, W.S. (1994). *S-PLUS Trellis Graphics User's Manual Version 3.3*. Mathsoft Inc., Seattle.

Begg, C.B. (1994). Publication bias, in H. Cooper and L.V. Hedges (eds), *The Handbook of Research Synthesis*. Russell Sage Foundation, New York.

Betemps, E.J. and Buncher, C.R. (1993). Birthplace as a risk factor in motor neurone disease and Parkinson's disease. *International Journal of Epidemiology* **22**, 898–904.

Biggerstaff, B.J. and Tweedie, R.L. (1997). Incorporating variables in estimates of heterogeneity in the random effects model in meta-analysis. *Statistics in Medicine* **16**, 753–768.

Blackstone, E.H., Naftel, D.C. and Turner, M.E. (1986). The decomposition of time varying hazard into phases, each incorporating a separate stream of concomitant information. *Journal of the American Statistical Association* **81**, 615–624.

Bland, M. (2000). *An Introduction to Medical Statistics*, 3rd edn. Oxford University Press, Oxford.

Breddin, K., Loew, D., Lechner, K. and Uberla, E.W. (1979). Secondary prevention of myocardial infarction. Comparison of acetylsalicylic acid, phenprocoumon and placebo. A multicenter two-year prospective study. *Thrombosis and Haemostasis* **41**, 225–236.

Breiman, L., Friedman, J.H., Olshen, R.A. and Stone, C.J. (1984). *Classification and Regression Trees*. Chapman & Hall, New York.

Breslow, N.E. (1974). Covariance analysis of censored survival data. *Biometrics* **30**, 89–99.

Breslow, N.E. and Day, N.E. (1980). *The Analysis of Case-Control Studies*. IARC Scientific Publications, Lyon, France.

Brown, B.W. (1980). Prediction analysis for binary data, in R.J. Miller, B. Efron, B.W. Brown and L.E. Moses (eds), *Biostatistics Casebook*. Wiley, New York.

Bullmore, E.T., Brammer, M.J., Williams, S.C.R., Rabe-Hesketh, S., Janot, W., David, A., Mellers, J., Howard, R. and Sham, P. (1996). Statistical methods of estimation and inference for functional MR image analysis. *Magnetic Resonance Medicine* **35**, 261–277.

Campbell, M.J. and Machin, D. (1999). *Medical Statistics: A Commonsense Approach*, 3rd edn. Wiley, Chichester.

Carpenter, J., Pocock, S. and Lamm, C.J. (2002) Coping with missing data in clinical trials: A model-based approach applied to asthma trials. *Statistics in Medicine* **21**, 1043–1066.

Chalmers, T.C. (1987). Meta-analysis in clinical medicine. *Transactions of the American Clinical Chematology Association* **99**, 144–150.

Chalmers, T.C. and Lau, J. (1993). Meta-analytic stimulus for changes in clinical trials. *Statistical Methods in Medical Research* **2**, 161–172.

Chambers, J.M. and Hastie, T.J. (1993). *Statistical Models in S*. Chapman & Hall, New York.

Choi, S.C., Muizelaar, J.P. and Barnes, T.Y. (1991). Prediction tree for severely head-injured patients. *Journal of Neurosurgery* **75**, 251–255.

Ciampi, A., Couturier, A. and Li, S. (2002) Prediction trees with soft nodes for binary outcomes. *Statistics in Medicine* **21**, 1145–1165.

Cleveland, W.S. (1979). Robust locally weighted regression and smoothing scatterplots. *Journal of the American Statistical Association* **74**, 829–836.

Cochran, W.G. (1954). Some methods for strengthening the common chi-square tests. *Biometrics* **10**, 417–451.

Colditz, G.A., Brewer, F.B., Berkey, C.S., Wilson, E.M., Burdick, E., Fineberg, H.V. and Mosteller, F. (1994). Efficacy of BCG vaccine in the prevention of tuberculosis. *Journal of the American Medical Association* **271**, 698–702.

Collett, D. (1991). *Modelling Binary Data*. Chapman & Hall, London.

Collett, D. (1994). *Modelling Survival Data in Medical Research*. Chapman & Hall, London.

Collett, D. and Jemain, A.A. (1985). Residuals, outliers, and influential observations in regression analysis. *Sains Malaysiana* **14**, 493–511.

Cook, R.D. and Weisberg, S. (1994). *Residuals and Influence in Regression*. Chapman & Hall, London.

Cook, R.J. (1998). Generalized linear model, in P. Armitage and T. Colton (eds), *Encyclopedia of Biostatistics*. Wiley, Chichester.

Copas, J.B. and Shi, J.Q. (2001). A sensitivity analysis for publication bias in systematic reviews. *Statistical Methods in Medical Research* **10**, 251–265.

Coronary Drug Project Group (1976). Coronary Drug Project Group. Aspirin in coronary heart disease. *Journal of Chronic Diseases* **29**, 625–642.

Cottingham, J. and Hunter, D. (1992). Chlamydia trachomatis and oral contraceptive use: a quantitative review. *Genitourinary Medicine* **68**, 209–216.

Cox, D.R. (1972). Regression models and life tables. *Journal of the Royal Statistical Society, Series B* **34**, 187–220.

Cramer, J.A., Collins, J.F. and Mallson, R.H. (1988). Can categorization of patient background problems be used to determine early termination in a clinical trial? *Controlled Clinical Trials* **9**, 47–63.

Daniel, W. (1995). *Biostatistics: A Foundation for Analysis in the Health Sciences,* 6th edn. Wiley, New York.

Daris, G.E., Applegate, W.B., Gordon, D.J., Curtis, C. and McCormick, M. (1995). An empirical evaluation of the placebo run-in. *Controlled Clinical Trials* **16**, 41–50.

Davis, C.S. (1991). Semi-parametric and non-parametric methods for the analysis of repeated measurements with applications to clinical trials. *Statistics in Medicine* **10**, 1959–1980.

Dawber, T.R. (1980). *The Framingham Study: The Epidemiology of Atherosclerotic Disease*. Harvard University Press, Cambridge, MA.

Dear, H.B.G. and Begg, C.B. (1992). An approach for assessing publication bias prior to performing a meta-analysis. *Statistical Science* **7**, 237–245.

DeMets, D.L. (1987). Methods for combining randomized clinical trials: strengths and limitations. *Statistics in Medicine* **6**, 341–348.

Der, G. and Everitt, B.S. (2001). *A Handbook of Statistical Analysis using SAS*, 2nd edn. Chapman & Hall/CRC, Boca Raton, FL.

Der Simonian, R. and Laird, N. (1986). Meta-analysis in clinical trials. *Controlled Clinical Trials* **7**, 177–188.

Diggle, P.J. (1998). Dealing with missing values in longitudinal studies, in B.S. Everitt and G. Dunn (eds), *Statistical Analysis of Medical Data*. Arnold, London.

Diggle, P.J. and Kenward, M.G. (1994). Informative dropout in longitudinal analysis (with discussion). *Applied Statistics* **43**, 49–93.

Diggle, P.J., Liang, K.Y. and Zeger, S.L. (1994). *Analysis of Longitudinal Data*. Oxford Scientific Publications, Oxford.

Dobson, A.J. (2001) *An Introduction to Generalized Linear Models*, 2nd edn. Chapman & Hall/CRC, Boca Raton, FL.

Dockery, D.W., Speizer, F.E., Strom, D.O., Ware, J.H., Spengler, J.D. and Ferns, B.G. (1989). Effects of inhalable particles on respiratory health in children. *American Review of Respiratory Disease* **139**, 587–597.

Duval, S. and Tweedie, R.L. (2000). A nonparametric 'trim and fill' method of accounting for publication bias in meta-analysis. *Journal of the American Statistical Association* **95**, 89–98.

Easterbrook, P.J., Berlin, J.A., Gepalas, R. and Matthews, D.R. (1991). Publication bias in research. *Lancet* **337**, 867–872.

Efron, B. (1998). Foreword in special issue on Analysing Non-Compliance in Clinical Trials. *Statistics in Medicine* **17**.

Efron, B. and Tibshirani, R.J. (1993). *An Introduction to the Bootstrap*. Chapman & Hall, London.

Egger, M., Smith, G.D., Schneider, M. and Minder, C. (1997). Bias in meta-analysis detected by a simple graphical test. *British Medical Journal* **315**, 629–634.

Elwood, P.C. and Sweetman, P.M. (1979). Aspirin and secondary mortality after myocardial infarction. *Lancet* **ii**, 1313–1315.

Elwood, P.C., Cochrane, A.L., Burr, M.L., Sweetman, P.M., Williams, G., Welsby, E., Hughes, S.J. and Renton, R. (1974). A randomized controlled trial of acetyl salicylic acid in the secondary prevention of mortality from myocardial infarction. *British Medical Journal* **1**, 436–440.

Everitt, B.S. (1996). An introduction to finite mixture distributions. *Statistical Methods in Medical Research* **5**, 107–127.

Everitt, B.S. (1998). *Cambridge Dictionary of Statistics*. Cambridge University Press, Cambridge.

Everitt, B.S. (2001a). *Statistics for Psychologists*. Lawrence Erlbaum, Mahwah, NJ.

Everitt, B.S. (2001b). *A Handbook of Statistical Analysis using S-PLUS*, 2nd Edn. Chapman & Hall/CRC, Boca Raton, FL.

Everitt, B.S. and Bullmore, E.T. (1999). Mixture model mapping of brain activation in functional magnetic resonance images. *Human Brain Mapping* **7**, 1–14.

Everitt, B.S. and Dunn, G. (2001). *Applied Multivariate Data Analysis*, 2nd edn. Arnold, London.

Everitt, B.S. and Hand, D.J. (1981). *Finite Mixture Distributions*. Chapman & Hall, London.

Everitt, B.S. and Pickles, A. (2000). *Statistical Aspects of the Design and Analysis of Clinical Trials*. Imperial College Press, London.

Everitt, B.S. and Rabe-Hesketh, S. (2001). *Analysing Medical Data using S-PLUS*. Springer, New York.

Everitt, B.S., Landau, S. and Leese, M. (2001). *Cluster Analysis*, 4th edn. Arnold, London.

Feinstein, A.R. (1991). Intention-to-treat policy for analysing randomized trials: Statistical distortions and neglected clinical challenges, in J.A. Cramer and B. Spilker (eds), *Patient Compliance in Medical Practice and Clinical Trials*. Raven Press Limited, New York.

Fergusson, D.M. and Horwood, L.J. (1989). A latent class model of smoking experimentation in children. *Journal of Child Psychology and Psychiatry* **30**, 761–773.

Fisher, L.D. and van Belle, G. (1993). *Biostatistics: A Methodology for the Health Sciences.* Wiley, New York.

Fisher, N.I. and Switzer, P. (1985). Chi-plots for assessing dependence. *Biometrika* **72,** 253–265.

Fisher, N.I. and Switzer, P. (2001). Graphical assessment of dependence: Is a picture worth 100 tests? *American Statistician* **55,** 233–239.

Fisher, R.A. (1935) *The Design of Experiments.* Oliver and Boyd, Edinburgh.

Ford, I. and Holmes, A.P. (1998). Functional neuroimaging and statistics, in B.S. Everitt and G. Dunn (eds), *Statistical Analysis of Medical Data.* Arnold, London.

Formann, A.K. and Kohlmann, T. (1996). Latent class analysis in medical research. *Statistical Methods in Medical Research* **5,** 179–211.

Freedman, L.S. and Spiegelhalter, D.J. (1983). The assessment of subjective opinion and its use in relation to stopping rules for clinical trials. *The Statistician* **32,** 153–161.

Freedman, L.S., Spiegelhalter, D.J. and Parmar, M.K.B. (1994). The what, why, and how of Bayesian clinical trials monitoring. *Statistics in Medicine* **13,** 1371–1384.

Friedman, J.H. (1991). Multiple adaptive regression splines. *Annals of Statistics* **19,** 1–67.

Friedman, L.M., Furberg, C.D. and DeMets, D.L. (1985). *Fundamentals of Clinical Trials,* 2nd edn. PSB Publishing, Littleton, MA.

Frierich, E., Gehan, E. *et al.* (1963). The effect of 6-mercaptopurine on the duration of steroid-induced remissions in acute leukaemia: a model for evaluation of other potentially useful therapies. *Blood* **21,** 699–716.

Gail, M.H., Lubin, J.H. and Rubinstein, L.V. (1981). Likelihood calculations for matched case-control studies and survival studies with tied death times. *Biometrika* **68,** 703–707.

Gared, A. (1988). Schizophrenia and birth complications. Unpublished manuscript.

Gelfand, A.E. and Smith, A.F.M. (1990). Sampling based approaches to calculating marginal densities. *Journal of the American Statistical Association* **85,** 398–409.

Geman, S. and Geman, D. (1984). Stochastic relaxation, Gilks distributions and the Bayesian restoration of images. *IEEE Transactions on Pattern Analysis and Machine Intelligence* **6,** 721–741.

Giardiello, F.M., Hamilton, S.R., Krush, A.J., Piantadosi, S., Hylind, L.M., Celano, P., Booker, S.V., Robinson, C.R. and Offerlaws, G.J.A. (1993). Treatment of colonic and rectal adenomas with sulindac in familial adenomatous polyposis. *New England Journal of Medicine* **328,** 1313–1316.

Gilks, W.R., Richardson, S. and Spiegelhalter, D.J. (eds) (1996). *Markov Chain Monte Carlo in Practice.* Chapman & Hall, London.

Givens, G.H., Smith, D.D. and Tweedie, R.L. (1997). Publication bias in meta-analysis: a Bayesian data-augmentation approach to account for issues exemplified in the passive smoking debate (with discussion). *Statistical Science* **12,** 244–245.

Goetghebeur, E.J. and Shapiro, S.H. (1996). Analysing non-compliance in clinical trials: ethical imperative or mission impossible? *Statistics in Medicine* **15,** 2813–2826.

Goldberg, K.M. and Iglewicz, B. (1992). Bivariate extensions of the boxplot. *Technometrics* **34,** 307–320.

Goldman, L., Weinberg, M., Weisberg, M., Olshen, R.A., Cook, E.F. and Sargent, R.K. *et al.* (1982). A computer protocol to predict myocardial infarction in emergency department patients with chest pain. *New England Journal of Medicine* **307,** 588–596.

Goldman, L., Cook, F., Johnson, P., Brand, D., Rosion, G. and Lee, T. (1996). Prediction of the need for intensive care in patients who come to emergency departments with acute chest pain. *New England Journal of Medicine* **334,** 1498–1504.

Goodman, L.A. (1974). Exploratory latent structure analysis using both identifiable and unidentifable models. *Biometrika* **61,** 215–231.

Gordon, N.H. (1990). Maximum likelihood estimation for mixtures of two Gompertz distributions when censoring occurs. *Communications in Statistics – Simulation and Computation* **19,** 733–747.

Greenwald, A.G. (1975). Consequences of prejudice against the null hypothesis. *Psychological Bulletin* **85,** 845–857.

Greenwood, M. and Yule, G.U. (1920) An inquiry into the nature of frequency-distributions of multiple happenings. *Journal of the Royal Statistical Society* **83,** 255.

Haberman, S. (1978). *Analysis of Qualitative Data, Volume 1.* Academic Press, New York.

Hardin, J.W. (2000). LogXact 4.1 for Windows. *American Statistician* **54,** 320–321.

Harrell, F.E. (2001). *Regression Modelling Strategies with Applications to Linear Models, Logistic Regression and Survival Analysis.* Springer, New York.

Harrington, D. and Fleming, T. (1982). A class of rank test procedures for censored survival data. *Biometrika* **69,** 553–566.

Hastie, T.J. and Tibshirani, R.J. (1990). *Generalized Additive Models.* Chapman & Hall, London.

Hedges, L.V. (1984). Estimation of effect size under non-random sampling: the effects of censoring studies yielding statistically insignificant mean differences. *Journal of Educational Statistics* **9,** 61–85.

Higgins, J.E. and Koch, G.G. (1997). Variable selection and generalized chi-square analysis of categorical data applied to a large cross-sectional occupational health survey. *International Statistical Review* **45,** 51–62.

Hirji, K.F. (1992). Exact distributions for polytomous data. *Journal of the American Statistical Association* **87,** 487–492.

Hirji, K.F., Tsiatis, A.A. and Mehta, C.R. (1989). Median unbiased estimation for binary data. *American Statistician* **43,** 7–11.

Hjalmarson, A., Elmfeldt, D., Herlitz, J., Holmberg, S., Nyberg, G., Ryden, L., Swedberg, K., Waagstein, F., Waldenstram, A., Vedin, A., Wedel, H., Wilhelmsen, L. and Wilhelmsson, C. (1981). A double blind trial of metoprolol in acute myocardial infarction – effects on mortality. *Circulation* **64,** 140.

Horton, N.J. and Lipstz, S.R. (1999). Review of software to fit generalized estimating equation regression models. *American Statistician* **53,** 160–169.

Horton, N.J. and Lipstz, S.R. (2000). Multiple imputation in practice: comparison of software packages for regression models with missing variables. *American Statistician* **55,** 244–254.

Hosmer, D.W. and Lemeshow, S. (1989). *Applied Logistic Regression.* Wiley, New York.

ISIS-2 Collaborative Group (1988). ISIS-2 Collaborative Group. Randomized trial of intravenous streptokinase, oral aspirin, both, or neither among 17,187 cases of suspected acute myocardial infarction: ISIS-2. *Lancet* **2,** 349–360.

Iyengar, S.I. and Greenhouse, J.B. (1988). Selection models and the file drawer problem. *Statistical Science* **3,** 109–117.

Jorgensen, M. and Hunt, L.A. (1999). Mixture model clustering using the MULTMIX program. *Australian and New Zealand Journal of Statistics* **41,** 153–171.

Kalbfleisch, J.D. and Prentice, R.L. (1980). *The Statistical Analysis of Failure Time Data.* Wiley, New York.

King, E.B., Chew, K.L., Petrakis, N.L. and Ernster, V.L. (1983). Nipple aspirate cytology for the study of breast cancer precursors. *Journal of the National Cancer Institute* **71,** 1115–1121.

Klein, J.P. and Moeschberger, M.L. (1997). *Survival Analysis.* Springer, New York.

Kraepelin, E. (1919). *Dementia Praecox and Paraphrenia.* Livingstone, Edinburgh.

Lazarsfield, P.L. and Henry, N.W. (1968). *Latent Structure Analysis.* Houghton Mifflin, Boston.

Le Fanu, J. (1999). *The Rise and Fall of Modern Medicine.* Abacus, London.

Levine, R.R.J. (1981). Sex differences in schizophrenia: timing or subtypes? *Psychological Bulletin* **90,** 432–444.

Levy, D.E., Caronna, J.J. and Singer, B.H. (1985). Predicting outcome from hypoxic-schemic coma. *Journal of the American Medical Association* **253,** 1420–1426.

Levy, P.S. and Stolte, K. (2000). Statistical methods in public health and epidemiology: a look at the recent past and projections for the next decade. *Statistical Methods in Medical Research* **9,** 41–56.

Liang, K.Y. and Zeger, S.L. (1986). Longitudinal data analysis using generalized linear models. *Biometrika* **73**, 13–22.

Lindsey, J.K. and Lambert, P. (1998). On the appropriateness of marginal models for repeated measurements in clincial trials. *Statistics in Medicine* **17**, 447–469.

Little, R.J.A. (1995). Modelling the drop-out mechanism in repeated measure studies. *Journal of the American Statistical Association* **90**, 1112–1121.

Liu, I.M. (1998). Breslow–Day test, in P. Armitage and T. Colton (eds), *Encyclopedia of Biostatistics*. Wiley, Chichester.

McConnochie, K.M., Roghmann, K.J. and Pasternack, J. (1993). Developing prediction rules and evaluating observing patterns using categorical clinical markers: two complimentary procedures. *Medical Decision Making* **13**, 130–142.

McCullagh, P. and Nelder, J.A. (1989). *Generalized Linear Models*, 2nd edn. Chapman & Hall, London.

McGiffin, D.C., O'Brien, M.F., Galbraith, A.J., McLachlan, G.J., Stafford, E.G., Gardiner, M.A.H., Pohlner, P.G., Early, L. and Kear, L. (1993) An analysis of risk factors for death and mode-specific death following aortic valve replacement using allograft, xenograft and mechanical valves. *Journal of Thoracic and Cardiovascular Surgery* 106, 895–911.

McLachlan, G. and Peel, D. (2000). *Finite Mixture Models*. Wiley, New York.

McLachlan, G.J. (1987). On bootstrapping the likelihood ratio test statistic for the number of components in a normal mixture. *Applied Statistics* **36**, 318–324.

McLachlan, G.J. and Basford, K.E. (1988). *Mixture Models: Inference and Applications to Clustering*. Marcel Dekker, New York.

McLachlan, G.J. and McGiffin, D.C. (1994). On the role of finite mixture models in survival analysis. *Statistical Methods in Medical Research* **3**, 211–226.

McLachlan, G.J., Peel, D., Basford, K.E. and Adams, P. (1998). *The EMMI software for the fitting of mixtures of normal and t-components*. http://www.maths.uq.edu.au/~gjm/emmix/paper.html.

Machin, D. (1994). Discussions of the what, why and how of Bayesian clinical trials monitoring. *Statistics in Medicine* **13**, 1385–1390.

Matthews, J.N.S. (1994). Discussion of Diggle and Kenward. *Applied Statistics* **43**, 49–93.

Mehta, C.R. and Patel, N.R. (1983). A network algorithm for performing Fisher's exact test in $r \times c$ contingency tables. *Journal of the American Statistical Association* **78**, 427–434.

Mehta, C.R. and Patel, N.R. (1996a). *StatXact 3 Manual*. Cytel Software Corporation, Cambridge, MA.

Mehta, C. and Patel, N. (1996b) *LogXact for Windows*. Cytel Software Corporation, Cambridge, MA.

Meinert, C.L. (1986). *Clinical Trials – Design, Conduct and Analysis*. Oxford University Press, New York.

Meir, P. (1987). Commentary. *Statistics in Medicine* **6**, 329–331.

Morgan, J.N. and Messenger, R.C. (1973) THAID: a sequential search program for analysis of nominal scale dependent variables. Technical report, Institute for Social Research, University of Michigan.

Morgan, J.N. and Sonquist, J.A. (1963). Problems in the analysis of survey data, and a proposal. *Journal of the American Statistical Association* **58**, 415–434.

Murray, G.D. and Findlay, J.G. (1988). Correcting for the bias caused by dropouts in hypertension trials. *Statistics in Medicine* **7**, 941–946.

Muthén, L.K. and Muthén, B.O. (1998). *Mplus Users Guide*. Muthén & Muthén, Los Angeles.

Nelder, J.A. and Wedderburn, R.W.M. (1972). Generalized linear models. *Journal of the Royal Statistical Society, Series A* **135**, 370–384.

Normand, S.T. (1999). Meta-analysis: formulating, evaluating, combining and reporting. *Statistics in Medicine* **18**, 321–359.

Pearson, K. (1894). Contributions to the theory of mathematical evolution, II: Skew variation. *Philosophical Transactions of the Royal Society of London, A* **186,** 343–414.

Peduzzi, P., Wittes, J. and Detre, K. (1993). Analysis as-randomized and the problem of non-adherence: an example from the Veterans Affairs Randomized Trial of Coronary Artery Bypass Surgery. *Statistics in Medicine* **12,** 1185–1195.

Peel, D. and McLachlan, G.J. (1999) *User's Guide to EMMIX.* http://www.maths.uq. edu.au/~gjm/emmix/emmix.html.

Persantine-Aspirin Reinfarction Study Research Group (1980). Persantine-Aspirin Reinfarction Study Research Group. Persantine and aspirin in coronary heart disease. *Circulation* **62,** 449–461.

Petitti, D.B. (2000). *Meta-analysis, Decision Analysis and Cost-Effectiveness Analysis.* Oxford University Press, New York.

Petrakis, N.L., Ernster, V.L., Sacks, S.T., King, E.B., Schweitzer, R.J., Hunt, T.K. and King, M.-C. (1981). Epidemiology of breast fluid secretion. Association with breast cancer risk factors and cerumen type. *Journal of the National Cancer Institute* **67,** 277–284.

Piantadosi, S. (1997). *Clinical Trials: A Methodologic Perspective.* Wiley, New York.

Pickering, R.M. and Forbes, J.F. (1984). A classification of Scottish infants using latent class analysis. *Statistics in Medicine* **3,** 249–259.

Pinheiro, J.C. and Bates, D.M. (2000). *Mixed-Effects Models in S and S-PLUS.* Springer, New York.

Rabe-Hesketh, S., Brammer, M.J. and Bullmore, E.T. (1998). Localizing brain activation in a single subject using functional magnetic resonance imaging, in B.S. Everitt and G. Dunn (eds), *Statistical Analysis of Medical Data.* Arnold, London.

Rabe-Hesketh, S. and Everitt, B.S. (2000). *A Handbook of Statistical Analysis using STATA,* 2nd edn. Chapman & Hall/CRC, Boca Raton, FL.

Roberts, G.O. (1996). Markov chain concepts related to sampling algorithms, in W.R. Gilks, S. Richardson and D.J. Spiegelhalter (eds), *Markov Chain Monte Carlo in Practice.* Chapman & Hall, London.

Robins, J.M., Rotnitzky, A. and Zhao, L.P. (1995). Analysis of semiparametric regression models for repeated outcomes in the presence of missing data. *Journal of the American Statistical Association* **90,** 106–121.

Rubin, D.B. (1976). Inference and missing data. *Biometrika* **63,** 581–592.

Schafer, J.L. (1999). Multiple imputation: a primer. *Statistical Methods in Medical Research* **8,** 3–16.

Schimert, J., Schafter, J.L., Hesterberg, T., Fraley, C. and Clarkson, D.B. (2000) *Analysing Data with Missing Values in S-PLUS.* Insightful Corporation, Seattle.

Schoenfeld, D.A. (1982). Partial residuals for the proportional hazards regression model. *Biometrika* **39,** 499–503.

Seeber, G.U.H. (1989). On the regression analysis of tumour recurrence rates. *Statistics in Medicine* **8,** 1363–1369.

Seeber, G.U.H. (1998). Poisson regression, in P. Armitage and T. Colton (eds), *Encyclopedia of Biostatistics.* Wiley, Chichester.

Segal, M.R. (1998). Tree-structured survival analysis in medical research, in B.S. Everitt and G. Dunn (eds), *Statistical Analysis of Medical Data.* Arnold, London.

Senchaudhuri, P., Mehta, C.R. and Patel, N.R. (1995). Estimating exact *p*-values by the method of control variates, or Monte Carlo rescue. *Journal of the American Statistical Association* **90,** 640–648.

Senn, S. (1997). *Statistical Issues in Drug Development.* Wiley, Chichester.

Silliman, N.P. (1997a). Nonparametric classes of weight functions to model publication bias. *Biometrika* **84,** 909–918.

Silliman, N.P. (1997b). Hierarchical selection models with applications in meta analysis. *Journal of the American Statistical Association* **92**, 926–936.

Silverman, B.W. (1986). *Density Estimation for Statistics and Data Analysis*. Chapman & Hall, London.

Skinner, C.J. (1994). Discussion of Diggle and Kenward. *Applied Statistics* **43**, 49–93.

Smith, M.L. (1980). Publication bias and meta-analysis. *Evaluating Education* **4**, 22–24.

Sockett, E.B., Daneman, D., Clarson, C., and Ehrich, R.M. (1987) Factors affecting and patterns of residual insulin secretion during the first year of Type I (insulin dependent) diabetes mellitus in children. *Diabet*, **30**, 453–459.

Spiegelhalter, D., Thomas, A., Best, N. and Gilks, W. (1996) BUGS 0.5 Examples, *Volume 1 (Version i)*. Cambridge: MRC Biostatistics Unit. http://www.mrc-bsu.cam.ac.uk/bugs/documentation/Download/eg05vol1.pdf.

Stanta, G. and Walker, A. (1986). Radiation and lung cancer. Technical paper, Harvard School of Public Health.

Sterlin, T.D. (1959). Publication decisions and their possible effects on inferences drawn from tests of significance – or vice versa. *Journal of the American Statistical Association* **54**, 30–34.

Stewart, L.A. and Parmar, M.K.B. (1993). Meta-analysis of the literature or of individual patient data: Is there a difference? *Lancet* **341**, 418–422.

Sutton, A.J. and Abrams, K.R. (2001). Bayesian methods in meta-analysis and evidence synthesis. *Statistical Methods in Medical Research* **10**, 277–303.

Sutton, A.J., Abrams, K.R., Jones, D.R. and Sheldon, T.A. (2000). *Methods for Meta-analysis in Medical Research*. Wiley, Chichester.

Talairach, J. and Tournoux, P. (1988). *A Coplanar Stereotoxic Atlas of the Human Brain*. Thieme-Verlag, Stuttgart.

Tanner, M.A. and Wong, W.H. (1987) The calculation of posterior distributions by data augmentation (with discussion). *Journal of the American Statistical Association* **82**, 528–550.

Tarone, R.E. and Ware, J. (1977). On distribution-free tests for equality of survival distributions. *Biometrika* **64**, 156–160.

Taylor, S.J. and Tweedie, R.L. (1998a). A parametric 'trim and fill' method of assessing publication bias in meta-analysis. Department of Statistics, Colorado State University.

Taylor, S.J. and Tweedie, R.L. (1998b). Trim and fill: a simple funnel plot based method of testing and adjusting for publication bias in meta-analysis. Department of Statistics, Colorado State University.

Temkin, N.R., Holubkov, R., Machamcer, J.E., Winn, H. and Dickme, S.S. (1995). Classification and regression trees (CART) for prediction of function at 1 year following head trauma. *Journal of Neurosurgery* **82**, 764–771.

Thall, P.F. and Vail, S.C. (1990). Some covariance models for longitudinal count data with overdispersion. *Biometrics* **46**, 657–671.

Therneau, T.M. and Grambsch, P.M. (2000). *Modeling Survival Data: Extending the Cox Model*. Springer, New York.

Trivedi, M.H. and Rush, H. (1994). Does a placebo run-in or a placebo treatment affect the efficacy of antidepressant medications? *Neuropsychopharmacology* **11**, 33–43.

Troxel, A.B., Fairclough, D.L., Curran, D. and Hahn, E.A. (1998). Statistical analysis of quality of life with missing data in cancer clinical trials. *Statistics in Medicine* **17**, 653–666.

Tufte, E.R. (1983). *The Visual Display of Quantitative Information*. Graphics Press, Cheshire, CT.

Urquhart, J. and de Klerk, E. (1998). Contending paradigms for the interpretation of data on patient compliance with therapeutic drug regimens. *Statistics in Medicine* **17**, 251–268.

Vaupel, J.W., Manton, K.G. and Stallard, E. (1979). The impact of heterogeneity in individual frailty on the dynamics of mortality. *Demography* **16**, 439–454.

Verbyla, A.P., Cullis, B.R., Kenward, M.G. and Welham, S.J. (1999). The analysis of designed experiments and longitudinal data using smoothing splines (with discussion). *Applied Statistics* **48**, 269–312.

Waldo, A.L., Camm, A.J., deRuyter, H. *et al.* (1996). Effect of d-sotalol on mortality in patients with left ventricular dysfunction after recent and remote myocardial infarction: the SWORD Investigators: Survival With Oral d-Sotalol. *Lancet* **348**, 7–12.

Ware, J.H., Dockery, D.W., Spiro, A., Speizer, F.E. and Ferns, B.G. (1984). Passive smoking, gas cooking and respirator health of children living in six cities. *American Review of Respiratory Disease* **129**, 366–374.

Waterhouse, D.M., Calzene, K.A., Mele, C. and Brenner, D.E. (1993). Adherence of oral tamoxifen: a comparison of patient self-report, pill count and microelectronic monitoring. *Journal of Clinical Oncology* **11**, 1189–1197.

Wedel, M. (2001). GLIMMIX: Software for estimating mixtures and mixtures of generalized linear models. *Journal of Classification* **18**, 129–135.

Wolfe, J.H. (1970). Pattern clustering by multivariate mixture analysis. *Multivariate Behavioral Research* **5**, 329–350.

Wrensch, M.R., Petrakis, N.L., King, E.B., Miike, R., Mason, L., Chew, K.L., Lee, M.M., Ernster, V.L., Hilton, J.F., Schweitzer, R., Goodson III, W.H. and Hunt, T.K. (1992). Breast cancer incidence in women with abnormal cytology in nipple aspirates of breast fluid. *American Journal of Epidemiology* **135**, 130–141.

Zeger, S.L. and Karim, M.R. (1991). Generalized linear model with random effects: a Gibbs sampling approach. *Journal of the American Statistical Association* **86**, 79–86.

Zeger, S.L. and Liang, K.Y. (1986). Longitudinal data analysis for discrete and continuous outcomes. *Biometrics* **42**, 121–130.

Zelen, M. (1971). The analysis of several 2×2 contingency tables. *Biometrika* **58**, 129–137.

Zhang, H. and Singer, B. (1999). *Recursive Partitioning in the Health Sciences*. Springer, New York.

Zhou, X.H., Perkins, A.J. and Hui, S.L. (1999). Comparisons of software packages for generalized linear multilevel models. *American Statistician* **53**, 282–290.

Index

Printed and bound by CPI Group (UK) Ltd, Croydon, CR0 4YY

27/10/2024

14580284-0003